FERTILITY CHALLENGE

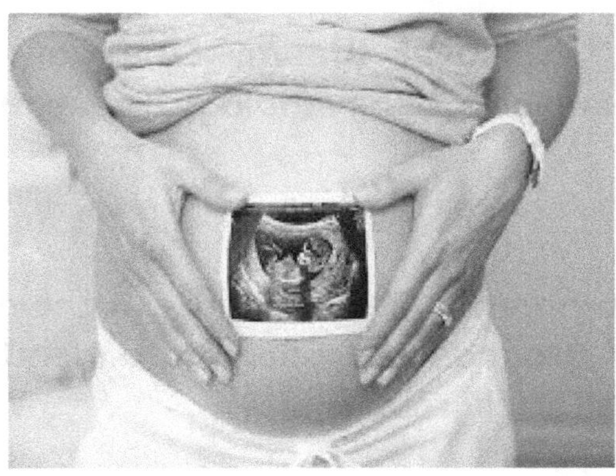

The intimate step by step guide about fertility challenges

TemmyPejju

Comprehensive Insight:** Uncover the mysteries of the mind as the book navigates through various facets of psychology, presenting a holistic view of the human experience.

Expert Guidance: Authored by seasoned psychologists and researchers, "Unlocking the Mind" is grounded in scientific understanding while remaining accessible to readers of all backgrounds.

Real-Life Stories: Engage with the narratives of individuals who have triumphed over mental challenges, demonstrating the resilience of the human spirit.

Practical Applications:** Gain valuable insights and practical tools to enhance your own mental well-being, fostering personal growth and self-awareness.
Timely Relevance: Addressing contemporary issues and trends in psychology, this book ensures that readers are equipped with knowledge that is both timeless and relevant

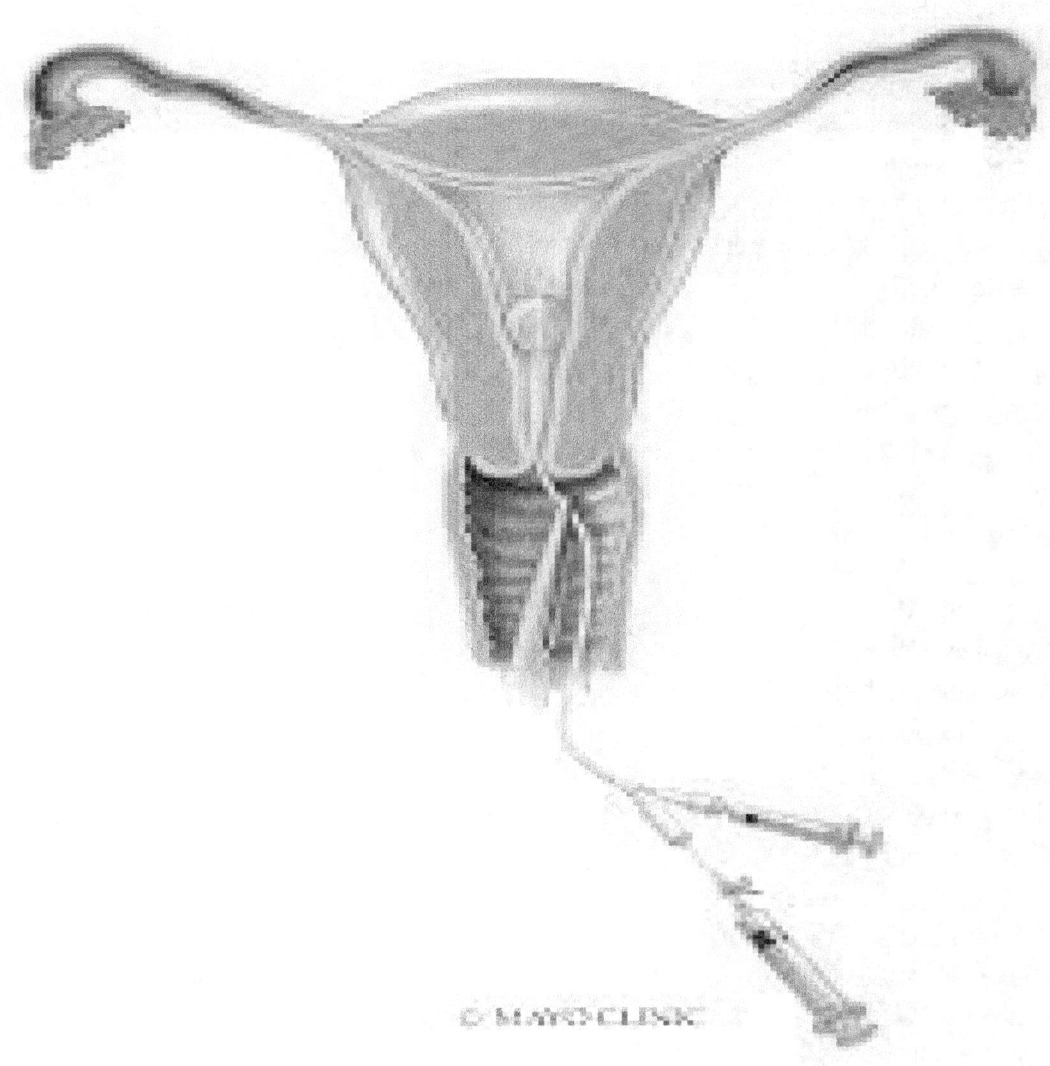

© MAYO CLINIC

Table of contents

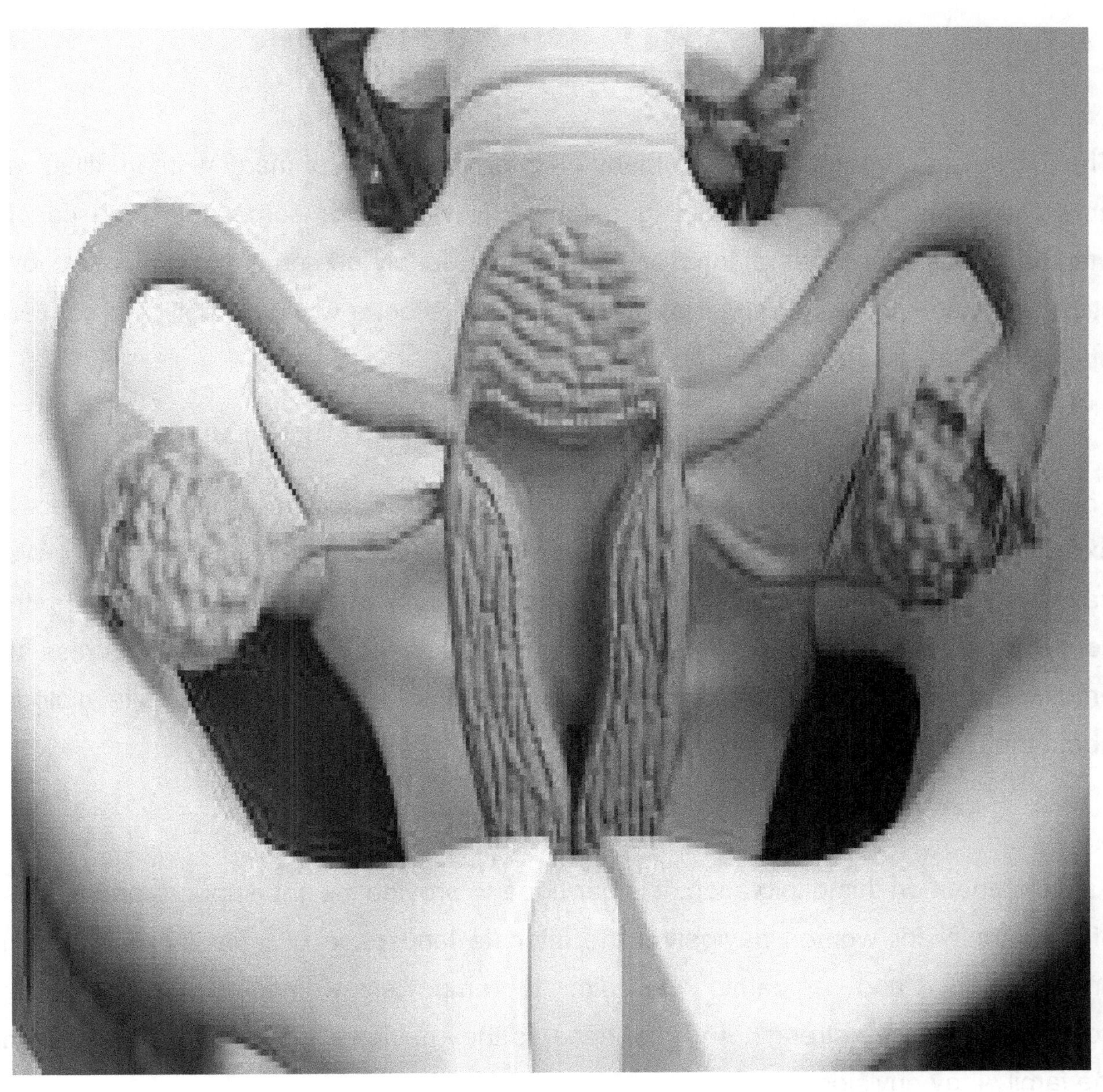

Introduction

The journey to parenthood is a profound chapter in the lives of many women, filled with anticipation and dreams of building a family. However, for some, this path can be marked by the challenges of infertility. Infertility, a deeply personal and often emotional struggle, encompasses a range of factors that can affect a woman's ability to conceive and carry a pregnancy to term.

This introduction delves into the complexities of infertility from a woman's perspective, exploring the biological, emotional, and societal dimensions of this intricate issue. We'll navigate the various causes, medical advancements, and holistic approaches that contribute to the broader understanding of infertility. Additionally, we'll address the emotional toll that infertility can take on women, fostering a compassionate dialogue about the unique challenges they face.

As we embark on this exploration, it is our hope to provide insight, support, and a sense of community for women navigating the intricate landscape of infertility. By fostering understanding and empathy, we aim to empower women on this journey, acknowledging their strength and resilience as they navigate the path towards creating the family they envision.

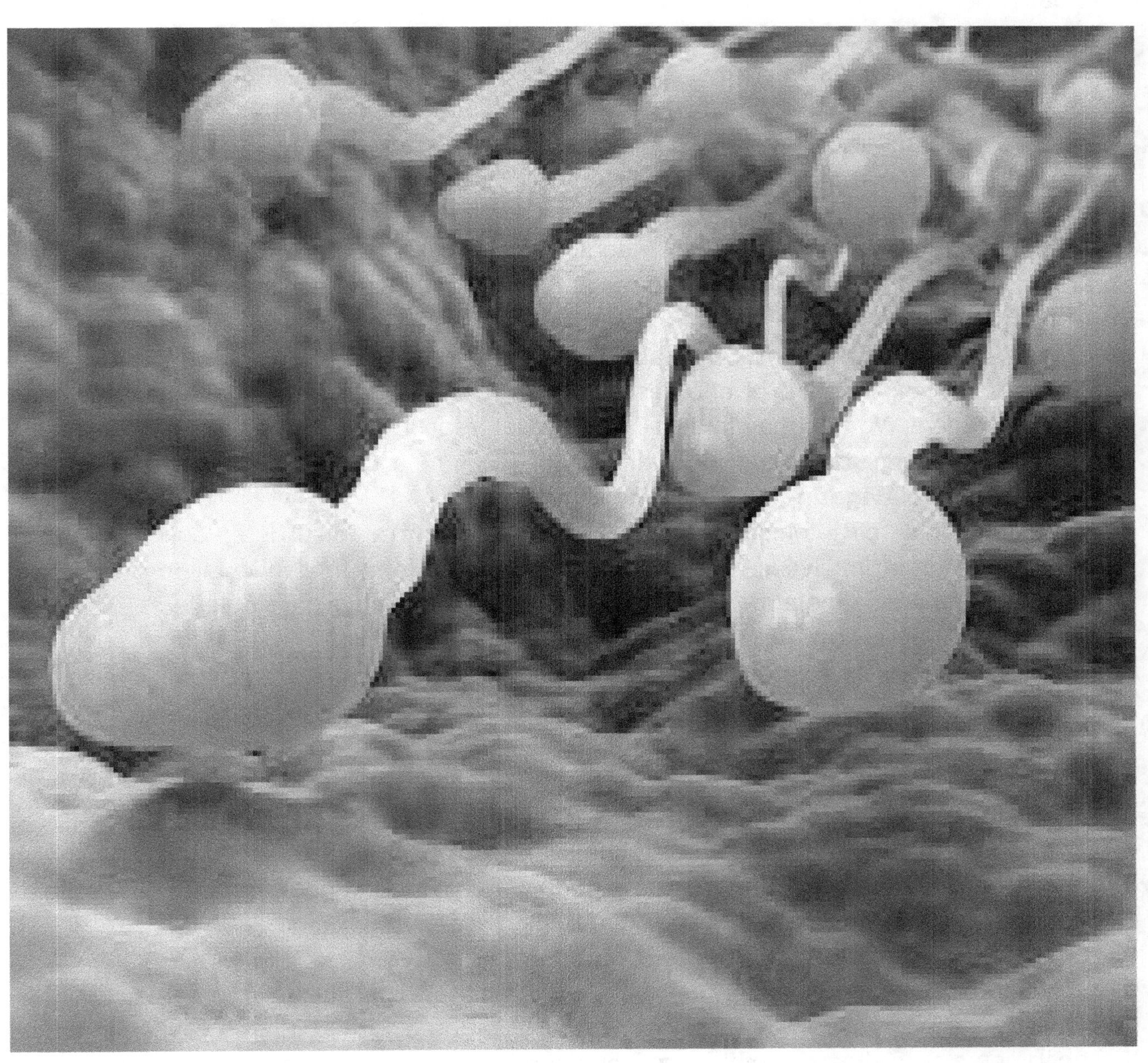

Chapter 1 The Emotional Landscape of Infertility

The emotional landscape of infertility is a terrain marked by a complex interplay of hope, despair, resilience, and often, unexpected twists. For many individuals and couples, the longing for a child becomes intertwined with the challenging reality of fertility struggles, creating a profound emotional journey that extends beyond medical diagnostics and treatments.

1. **Hope and Anticipation**:

Infertility often begins with hope and anticipation, as individuals embark on the journey of conceiving a child. Optimism and excitement are palpable, driven by the desire to expand one's family and embrace the joys of parenthood.

2. **Disappointment and Grief:**

As months pass without a successful conception, hope can transform into disappointment and grief. Each negative pregnancy test or unsuccessful fertility treatment can bring a wave of sadness and mourning for the envisioned family that has yet to materialize.

3. **Isolation and Stigma**:

The societal expectation of effortless conception can lead to feelings of isolation and stigmatization. Women may internalize a sense of failure, compounded by the pressure to conform to societal norms surrounding family planning.

4. **Navigating Medical Interventions:**

The emotional toll intensifies with the introduction of medical interventions. Fertility treatments often involve a rollercoaster of emotions, from the anticipation of potential success to the disappointment of setbacks and the toll of physical side effects.

5. **Relationship Dynamics**:

Infertility can strain relationships, as couples grapple with the emotional challenges together. Communication becomes pivotal, and navigating the emotional ups and downs requires mutual support, understanding, and sometimes seeking professional counseling.

6. **Coping Mechanisms**:

Individuals often develop coping mechanisms to manage the emotional burden. This might involve seeking support from friends, family, or support groups, as well as engaging in activities that bring solace and distraction.

7. **Decision-Making and Acceptance:**

The journey of infertility may lead to profound decision-making moments, such as considering alternative paths to parenthood or embracing a child-free life. Acceptance becomes a crucial aspect of the emotional landscape, fostering resilience and the ability to redefine one's vision of family.

8.   **Empowerment and Advocacy:**
As awareness about infertility grows, individuals often find empowerment in advocacy and education. Sharing experiences and dispelling myths can help break down societal stigmas, fostering a sense of community and support.

9.   **Embracing Resilience:**
Ultimately, the emotional landscape of infertility is a testament to the resilience of individuals and couples facing this challenge. It calls for acknowledging the strength needed to endure the emotional highs and lows, embracing hope, and finding fulfillment on a path that may deviate from conventional expectations.

In recognizing the emotional complexity of infertility, we aim to foster understanding, empathy, and support for individuals navigating this intricate landscape.

Understanding the Complexity of Fertility Challenges

Fertility challenges encompass a nuanced interplay of biological, emotional, and societal factors, rendering the journey to conception intricate and multifaceted. This section explores the diverse dimensions that contribute to the complexity of fertility challenges, shedding light on the myriad factors that individuals and couples may encounter.

1.   **Biological Factors:**
      Exploring Reproductive Anatomy
      Hormonal Influences on Fertility
      Impact of Age on Fertility

2.   **Common Causes and Conditions:**
      Unexplained Infertility
    Polycystic Ovary Syndrome (PCOS)
    Endometriosis
    Male Factor Infertility

3.   **Genetic Considerations:**
      Genetic Testing and its Role
    Inherited Fertility Conditions

4. **Environmental and Lifestyle Influences:**
Effects of Diet and Nutrition
. Impact of Stress on Fertility
Environmental Toxins and Fertility
5. **Reproductive Health Disparities:**
Addressing Disparities in Access to
Fertility Care
Cultural and Societal Influences on Reproductive Health
6. **Diagnostic Procedures:**
Fertility Testing for Men and Women
Imaging and Laboratory Techniques
7. **Assisted Reproductive Technologies (ART):** . In Vitro Fertilization (IVF)
Intracytoplasmic Sperm Injection (ICSI)
Egg and Sperm Donation
8. **Fertility Treatments and Options:**
Ovulation Inductio.
Intrauterine Insemination (IUI.

Surgical Interventions for Fertility
Understanding the complexity of fertility challenges necessitates a comprehensive exploration of these various facets. By delving into the biological intricacies, medical advancements, and societal influences surrounding fertility, individuals and couples can gain a more informed perspective on their unique journey. This knowledge lays the foundation for informed decision-making, empowers individuals to seek appropriate support, and fosters a more inclusive and understanding conversation about fertility challenges in society.

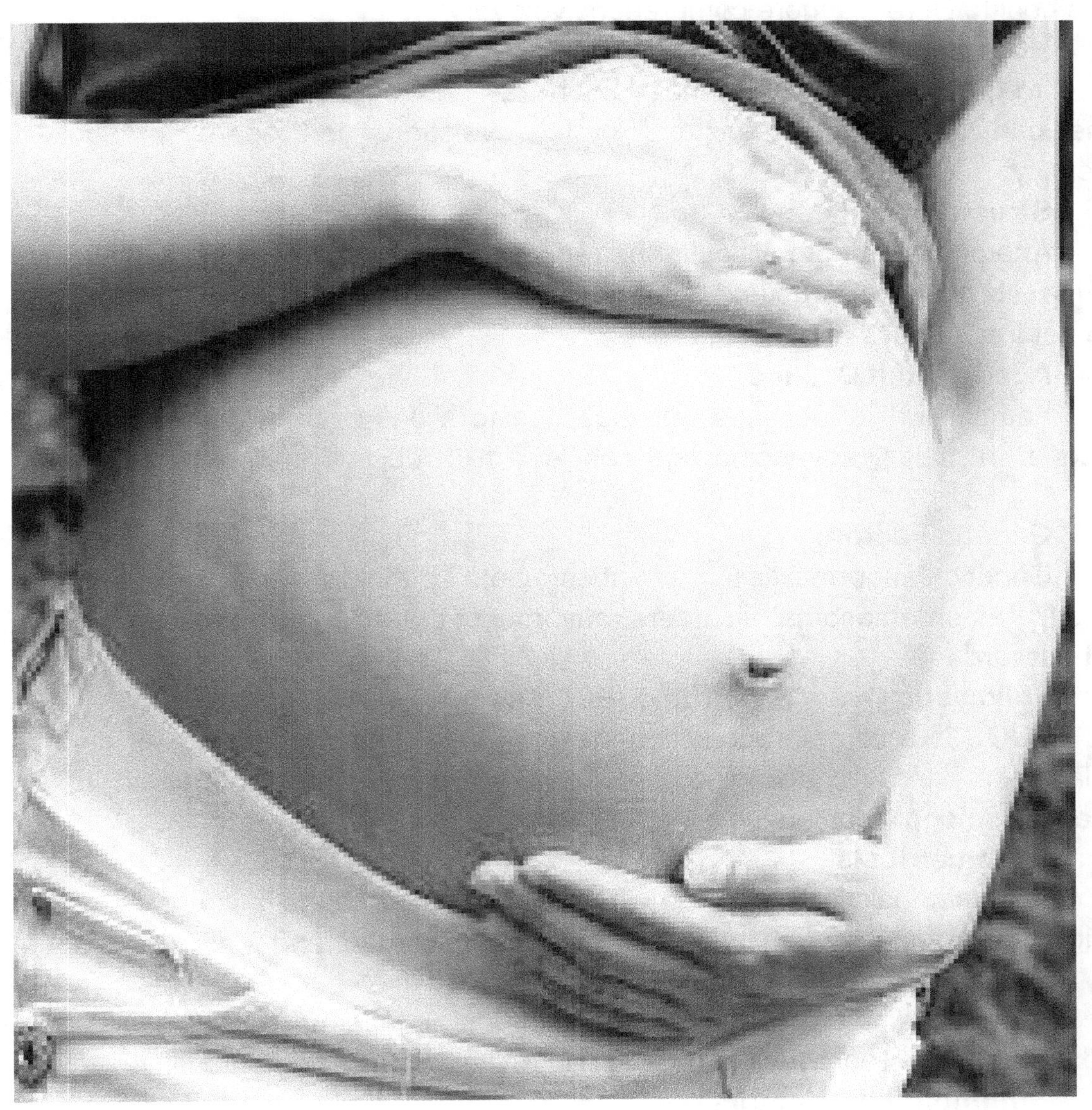

Chapter 2 Exploring Causes

Biological Factors

Biological factors affecting fertility are multifaceted and encompass various aspects of reproductive health. Here's a more comprehensive overview:

1. **Hormonal Imbalances**:
*   Irregularities in hormones such as estrogen, progesterone, and testosterone can disrupt the menstrual cycle, ovulation, and sperm production, hindering fertility.

2. **Structural Issues**:
*   Anatomical abnormalities in the reproductive organs, like blocked fallopian tubes, uterine fibroids, or structural defects in the male reproductive system, can impede the natural process of conception.

3. **Age-Related Decline**:
*   Female fertility declines with age due to a decrease in the quantity and quality of eggs. In males, advancing age can lead to a decline in sperm quality and motility.

4. **Genetic Factors**:
*   Genetic abnormalities can affect both partners, influencing fertility. Conditions such as chromosomal disorders may impact the ability to conceive or result in recurrent miscarriages.

5. **Polycystic Ovary Syndrome (PCOS)**:
*   PCOS is a common condition in women that can cause irregular periods and anovulation, making it challenging to conceive. It is often associated with insulin resistance and hormonal imbalances.

6. **Endometriosis**:
*   Endometriosis is a condition where tissue similar to the lining of the uterus grows outside the uterus. This can lead to inflammation, scarring, and fertility issues.

7. **Sexually Transmitted Infections (STIs)**:
*   Some STIs, if left untreated, can cause pelvic inflammatory disease (PID), leading to damage to the reproductive organs and an increased risk of infertility.

8. **Immunological Factors**:
*   Immune system disorders may affect fertility by causing the body to perceive sperm, eggs, or embryos as foreign, leading to an immune response that hampers conception.

9.   **Weight and Nutrition**:
•   Both underweight and overweight conditions can impact fertility. Extreme body weight changes can disrupt hormonal balance, affecting ovulation and sperm production.
10.   **Lifestyle Factors**:
•   Unhealthy lifestyle choices such as smoking, excessive alcohol consumption, and illicit drug use can adversely affect fertility in both men and women.
11.   **Stress**:
•   Chronic stress may impact reproductive hormones and disrupt the menstrual cycle, potentially affecting fertility.
Understanding these biological factors is crucial for individuals and couples facing fertility challenges. Seeking medical guidance and intervention can help identify specific issues and develop tailored approaches to address them.

Lifestyle and Environmental Influences

Lifestyle and environmental factors play a significant role in fertility challenges, affecting both men and women. Here's a comprehensive overview:
1.   **Nutrition and Diet**:
•   Poor nutrition and unhealthy eating habits can impact fertility. Nutrient deficiencies may affect reproductive hormones and ovulation in women, while in men, it can lead to lower sperm quality.
2.   **Body Weight and Exercise**:
•   Both underweight and overweight conditions can disrupt hormonal balance, affecting menstrual cycles in women and sperm production in men. Intense exercise, especially in women, may also influence fertility.
3.   **Smoking**:
•   Smoking has been linked to decreased fertility in both men and women. It can affect egg quality, sperm motility, and increase the risk of miscarriage.
4.   **Alcohol Consumption**:
•   Excessive alcohol intake can disrupt hormone levels and impair reproductive function. It may contribute to irregular menstrual cycles in women and reduce sperm quality in men.
5.   **Illicit Drug Use**:
•   Drug abuse, including the use of recreational drugs, can adversely impact fertility. It may disrupt hormonal balance and impair the development of healthy eggs and sperm.
6.   **Caffeine Intake**:

- While research is inconclusive, high caffeine intake has been associated with a slightly increased risk of fertility issues. It may affect female reproductive function and conception.

7. **Environmental Toxins:**
- Exposure to environmental pollutants, pesticides, and industrial chemicals may have endocrine-disrupting effects, influencing fertility by affecting hormone production and function.

8. **Heat Exposure**:
- Prolonged exposure to high temperatures, such as in hot tubs or saunas, may temporarily reduce sperm production in men, impacting fertility.

9. **Radiation**:
- Exposure to excessive radiation, whether from medical procedures or occupational sources, can harm reproductive organs and affect fertility.

10. **Work-Related Stress**:
- High levels of stress at work or in personal life can contribute to fertility challenges by disrupting hormonal balance and affecting menstrual cycles in women and sperm production in men.

11. **Plastic Chemicals (Phthalates):**
- Some chemicals found in plastics, like phthalates, have been associated with fertility issues. These substances may have endocrine-disrupting properties.

12. **Social and Economic Factors**:
- Socioeconomic factors, including access to healthcare, education, and economic stability, can indirectly influence fertility by affecting lifestyle choices and stress levels.

Understanding and addressing these lifestyle and environmental factors are essential for individuals or couples facing fertility challenges. Adopting healthier habits, seeking medical advice, and making informed lifestyle choices can contribute to improved reproductive health.

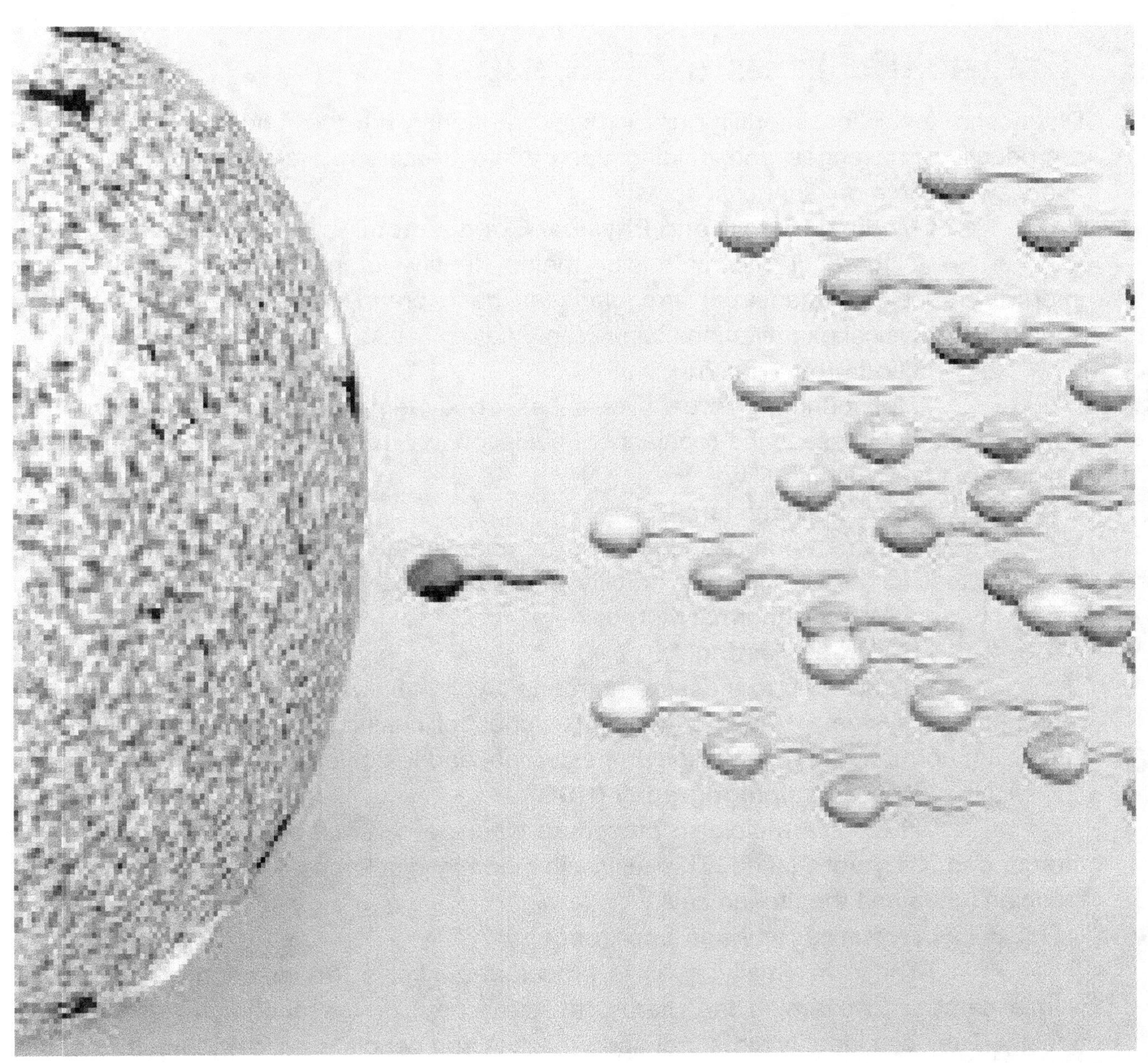

Chapter 3. Medical Perspectives

Diagnostic Tests for Infertility

Diagnostic tests for infertility are crucial in identifying the underlying causes of reproductive challenges and guiding appropriate treatment. Here's a comprehensive overview of common diagnostic tests:

1. **Medical History and Physical Examination:**
    *   A thorough medical history helps identify potential factors contributing to infertility, such as menstrual irregularities, past pregnancies, or existing health conditions. Physical examinations can reveal anatomical issues or abnormalities.
2. **Ovulation Tracking**:
    *   Monitoring menstrual cycles, basal body temperature, and using ovulation predictor kits help assess the regularity of ovulation in women. Lack of ovulation can be a significant factor in infertility.
3. **Semen Analysis:**
    *   A semen analysis evaluates the quantity, quality, and motility of sperm. It is a key test for assessing male fertility and can identify issues such as low sperm count, poor motility, or abnormal morphology.
4. **Hormone Testing**:
    *   Blood tests to measure hormone levels help assess the functioning of the reproductive system. Key hormones include follicle-stimulating hormone (FSH), luteinizing hormone (LH), estradiol, progesterone, and testosterone.
5. **Hysterosalpingography (HSG):**
    *   HSG is a radiologic procedure where a contrast dye is injected into the uterus, and X-rays are taken. This test helps identify blockages or abnormalities in the fallopian tubes and the uterine cavity.
6. **Hysteroscopy and Laparoscopy:**
    *   These minimally invasive procedures involve the insertion of a thin tube with a camera to examine the uterus (hysteroscopy) or the abdomen (laparoscopy) directly. They can identify structural abnormalities and conditions like endometriosis.
7. **Transvaginal Ultrasound**:
    *   This imaging technique uses sound waves to create images of the reproductive organs. It helps identify structural issues, such as ovarian cysts, fibroids, or polyps, and can assess the thickness of the uterine lining.

8.   **Genetic Testing**:
•   Genetic tests may be recommended to identify chromosomal abnormalities or genetic disorders that could impact fertility. This is particularly relevant for recurrent miscarriages or a family history of genetic conditions.

9.   **Anti-Mullerian Hormone (AMH) Test:**
•   AMH levels indicate ovarian reserve, providing insight into the quantity of remaining eggs. Low AMH levels may suggest a reduced ovarian reserve, affecting fertility.

10.   **Thyroid Function Tests:**
•   Thyroid disorders can impact fertility. Blood tests to assess thyroid function, including levels of thyroid-stimulating hormone (TSH) and thyroid hormones (T3 and T4), help diagnose and manage thyroid-related fertility issues.

11.   **Postcoital Test**:
•   This test evaluates the interaction between sperm and cervical mucus shortly after intercourse, providing insights into sperm viability and the cervical environment.

12.   **Endometrial Biopsy**:
•   An endometrial biopsy may be performed to assess the uterine lining for abnormalities or signs of inadequate receptivity for embryo implantation.

13.   **Immunological Tests**:
•   In some cases, immune system disorders may contribute to fertility challenges. Immunological tests can help identify any immune-related factors impacting fertility.

These diagnostic tests, often conducted in combination, enable healthcare professionals to tailor fertility treatments based on the specific issues identified, improving the chances of successful conception.

Assisted Reproductive Technologies (ART)

Assisted Reproductive Technologies (ART) encompass a range of medical procedures designed to aid couples and individuals in overcoming infertility. These advanced techniques aim to facilitate conception when natural methods prove unsuccessful. Here's a comprehensive overview of ART:

1.   **In Vitro Fertilization (IVF)**:
•   IVF involves combining eggs and sperm outside the body in a laboratory dish. Fertilized embryos are then transferred to the uterus. It's a versatile technique

used for various infertility causes, including tubal blockages, male factor infertility, and unexplained infertility.

2.   **Intracytoplasmic Sperm Injection (ICSI):**

•   ICSI involves the injection of a single sperm directly into an egg. This method is particularly useful in cases of severe male infertility or when previous IVF attempts have failed.

3.   **Gamete Intrafallopian Transfer (GIFT):**

•   GIFT involves placing eggs and sperm into the fallopian tubes, allowing fertilization to occur inside the body. This method is less common than IVF and is typically used in cases where tubal function is preserved.

4.   **Zygote Intrafallopian Transfer (ZIFT):**

•   ZIFT combines elements of IVF and GIFT. Fertilized embryos are transferred to the fallopian tubes rather than the uterus, aiming for natural fertilization within the body.

5.   **Frozen Embryo Transfer (FET):**

•   In FET, cryopreserved embryos from a previous IVF cycle are thawed and transferred to the uterus in a subsequent cycle. This allows for multiple attempts at conception without the need for a full IVF cycle.

6.   **Egg Donation:**

•   Egg donation involves using eggs from a donor for fertilization. This option is suitable for women with diminished ovarian reserve or those unable to produce viable eggs. The recipient undergoes IVF with the donor's eggs.

7.   **Sperm Donation:**

•   Sperm donation is used when male factor infertility is a concern. Donor sperm is used for fertilization through IUI or IVF. This option is chosen when the male partner has low sperm count, poor motility, or genetic concerns.

8.   **Surrogacy:**

•   Surrogacy involves a woman carrying and delivering a baby for another individual or couple. This method is used when a woman is unable to carry a pregnancy to term due to medical reasons.

9.   **Preimplantation Genetic Testing (PGT):**

•   PGT includes Preimplantation Genetic Screening (PGS) and Preimplantation Genetic Diagnosis (PGD). PGS examines embryos for chromosomal abnormalities, while PGD focuses on specific genetic disorders. This helps select healthy embryos for implantation.

10.   **Embryo Cryopreservation:**

• Embryo cryopreservation involves freezing and storing embryos for future use. This is often done in conjunction with IVF to preserve excess embryos for potential later transfers.

11. **Assisted Hatching**:

• Assisted hatching involves creating a small opening in the outer layer of the embryo (zona pellucida) to facilitate embryo implantation. It may be used in specific cases to enhance the chances of successful implantation.

12. **Ovulation Induction and Controlled Ovarian Stimulation:**

• These techniques involve using medications to stimulate the ovaries and promote the development of multiple eggs, increasing the chances of successful fertilization during ART procedures.

Assisted Reproductive Technologies have revolutionized fertility treatments, offering hope to individuals and couples facing challenges in conceiving naturally. The selection of a specific ART method depends on the underlying causes of infertility and the unique circumstances of each individual or couple.

Fertility Treatments and Options

Fertility treatments and options encompass a range of medical interventions aimed at assisting individuals and couples in achieving pregnancy. Here's a comprehensive guide covering various fertility treatments:

1. **Lifestyle Modifications**:

• Before considering medical interventions, adopting a healthy lifestyle is crucial. This includes maintaining a balanced diet, regular exercise, avoiding smoking and excessive alcohol consumption, and managing stress.

2. **Ovulation Induction**:

• Medications like Clomiphene citrate or letrozole stimulate ovulation in women who have irregular or absent menstrual cycles. This can enhance the chances of conception.

3. **Intrauterine Insemination (IUI):**

• IUI involves placing prepared sperm directly into the uterus during the woman's fertile window. It's a less invasive option, often used in cases of mild male factor infertility or unexplained infertility.

4. **In Vitro Fertilization (IVF):**

• IVF is a highly effective fertility treatment where eggs and sperm are combined outside the body, and resulting embryos are transferred to the uterus. It is suitable for various infertility causes, including tubal issues, endometriosis, and advanced maternal age.

5. **Intracytoplasmic Sperm Injection (ICSI):**
• ICSI is often used in conjunction with IVF. It involves injecting a single sperm directly into an egg, making it an effective solution for severe male infertility or previous IVF failures.

6. **Gamete Intrafallopian Transfer (GIFT):**
• GIFT involves placing eggs and sperm directly into the fallopian tubes to allow natural fertilization within the body. It's a less common option compared to IVF.

7. **Zygote Intrafallopian Transfer (ZIFT):**
• ZIFT combines elements of IVF and GIFT. Fertilized embryos are transferred to the fallopian tubes instead of the uterus.

8. **Egg Donation:**
• Egg donation is suitable for women with diminished ovarian reserve or those unable to produce viable eggs. It involves using eggs from a donor for fertilization through IVF.

9. **Sperm Donation:**
• Sperm donation is employed when male factor infertility is a concern. Donor sperm is used for fertilization through IUI or IVF.

10. **Surrogacy:**
• Surrogacy involves another woman carrying and delivering a baby for individuals or couples unable to carry a pregnancy. It may involve using the intended parents' genetic material or donor gametes.

11. **Preimplantation Genetic Testing (PGT):**
• PGT includes Preimplantation Genetic Screening (PGS) and Preimplantation Genetic Diagnosis (PGD). PGS examines embryos for chromosomal abnormalities, while PGD focuses on specific genetic disorders.

12. **Cryopreservation:**
• Embryo, egg, or sperm cryopreservation allows the freezing and storage of reproductive cells for future use. This is often done in conjunction with IVF.

13. **Assisted Hatching:**
• Assisted hatching involves creating a small opening in the outer layer of the embryo to facilitate implantation. It may be used in specific cases during IVF.

14. **Ovum (Egg) Freezing:**
• Women can opt to freeze their eggs for future use, preserving fertility, especially for those facing medical treatments that may impact ovarian function.

15. **Adoption:**

• Adoption is a non-biological option for building a family. It involves legally adopting and raising a child who is not biologically related to the adopting parents.

Choosing the most suitable fertility treatment involves a careful assessment of the underlying causes of infertility, the age of the individuals involved, and ethical, emotional, and financial considerations. Consulting with a fertility specialist is essential to explore personalized options and create a tailored treatment plan.

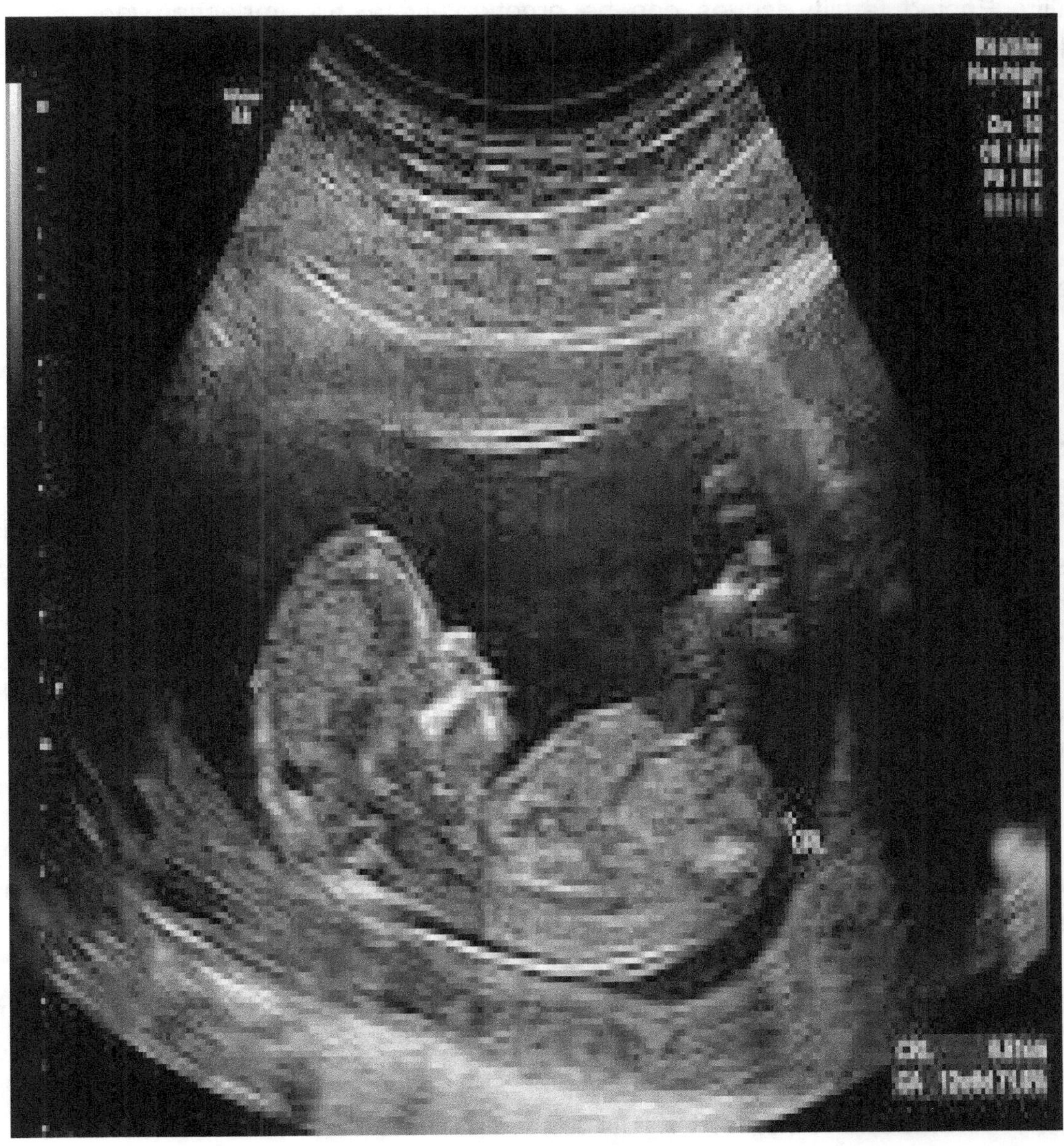

Chapter 4. Emotional Well-being

Emotional well-being is a critical aspect of navigating the challenges associated with infertility. Facing fertility issues can be emotionally taxing, impacting individuals and couples on various levels. Here's a concise overview of considerations for maintaining emotional well-being during infertility:

1.   **Acknowledge Emotions**:
•   It's essential to recognize and accept the range of emotions that may arise, including sadness, frustration, and anxiety. Allow yourself the space to feel and express these emotions.

2.   **Open Communication**:
•   Maintain open and honest communication with your partner. Infertility can strain relationships, and sharing feelings and concerns can foster understanding and support.

3.   **Seek Professional Support**:
•   Engaging with a mental health professional, such as a therapist or counselor, can provide a safe space to explore and manage the emotional impact of infertility.

4.   **Join Support Groups**:
•   Connecting with others experiencing similar challenges through support groups or online forums can offer a sense of community, shared understanding, and valuable coping strategies.

5.   **Set Realistic Expectations**:
•   Understand that the fertility journey can be unpredictable, and outcomes may not always align with expectations. Setting realistic goals and timelines can help manage disappointment.

6.   **Self-Care**:
•   Prioritize self-care activities that promote mental and emotional well-being, such as exercise, meditation, or hobbies. Taking breaks from fertility-related stressors is crucial.

7.   **Educate Yourself**:
•   Knowledge about fertility treatments, options, and potential outcomes can empower individuals and reduce feelings of uncertainty. Stay informed but also allow yourself breaks from constant research.

8.   **Establish Boundaries**:

- Set boundaries regarding discussions about fertility with others. It's okay to decide when and with whom you want to share information and when you need personal space.

9. **Celebrate Milestones**:
- Acknowledge and celebrate non-fertility-related achievements and milestones in your life. Focusing on other aspects can provide a sense of accomplishment and balance.

10. **Coping Strategies**:
- Develop healthy coping mechanisms, such as journaling, mindfulness, or engaging in activities that bring joy. Find what works best for you to manage stress.

11. **Empowerment and Advocacy:**
- Take an active role in your fertility journey. Advocate for yourself, ask questions, and collaborate with your healthcare team to make informed decisions.

12. **Explore Alternatives**:
- Be open to exploring alternative paths to parenthood, such as adoption or surrogacy. Flexibility in considering various options can alleviate some emotional stress.

13. **Embrace Positive Changes**:
- Focus on positive lifestyle changes that can enhance overall well-being. This might include improving nutrition, incorporating exercise, and fostering a supportive social network.

Remember that emotional well-being is a dynamic process, and seeking help when needed is a sign of strength. Infertility can be a challenging journey, but with emotional support and coping strategies, individuals and couples can navigate it more resiliently.

Coping with the Emotional Impact

Coping with the emotional impact of infertility is a deeply personal and challenging journey. Here's a comprehensive guide to help navigate the emotional aspects of fertility struggles:

1. **Acknowledge and Validate Emotions:**
- Accept the range of emotions you may experience, including grief, frustration, sadness, and anxiety. Understand that these feelings are valid responses to a challenging situation.

2. **Open Communication with Partner**:

- Maintain open and honest communication with your partner. Share your feelings, fears, and hopes. Jointly navigating the emotional aspects can strengthen the relationship.

3. **Educate Yourself**:
- Gain a thorough understanding of the fertility process, potential causes of infertility, and available treatments. Knowledge empowers individuals to make informed decisions and reduces anxiety.

4. **Seek Professional Support**:
- Consult with a mental health professional experienced in fertility issues. Therapy provides a safe space to express emotions, learn coping strategies, and receive support.

5. Join Support Groups:
- Connect with others facing infertility through support groups, both in-person and online. Sharing experiences with those who understand can provide comfort and reduce feelings of isolation.

6. **Set Realistic Expectations**:
- Understand that fertility treatments may not always result in immediate success. Set realistic expectations, recognizing that the journey may involve setbacks and unforeseen challenges.

7. **Self-Care Practices**:
- Prioritize self-care to manage stress. Engage in activities that bring joy, relaxation, and fulfillment, whether it's exercise, meditation, creative pursuits, or spending time in nature.

8. **Limit Fertility-Related Stress**:
- Establish boundaries concerning discussions about fertility with friends and family. Decide when and with whom you want to share information, allowing yourself breaks from constant fertility-related conversations.

9. **Celebrate Non-Fertility Achievements:**
- Acknowledge and celebrate achievements unrelated to fertility. Focusing on personal and professional successes can provide a sense of accomplishment and balance.

10. **Coping Strategies**:
- Develop healthy coping mechanisms, such as journaling, mindfulness, or engaging in activities that bring comfort. Identify what works best for you to manage stress and emotional challenges.

11. **Empowerment and Advocacy**:
- Take an active role in your fertility journey. Advocate for yourself, ask questions, and actively participate in decisions regarding treatment options.

12. **Consider Alternative Paths**:

- Be open to exploring alternative paths to parenthood, such as adoption, surrogacy, or embracing a child-free life. Flexibility in considering various options can provide a sense of empowerment.

13. **Embrace Support from Loved Ones:**

- Allow yourself to lean on friends and family for support. Share your feelings and let them know how they can best provide comfort during this challenging time.

14. **Focus on the Present Moment:**

- Practice mindfulness and stay present. Dwelling too much on the past or worrying about the future can contribute to heightened stress levels.

15. **Professional Guidance for Decision-Making:**

- Seek guidance from fertility specialists to make informed decisions about treatment options. Understanding the potential risks and benefits can help alleviate some uncertainty.

Coping with infertility is a unique and individual journey. Combining self-care practices, professional support, and open communication can contribute to emotional well-being and resilience throughout the fertility process.

Nurturing Mental Health during Fertility Struggles

Nurturing mental health during fertility struggles is crucial for overall well-being. The emotional toll of infertility can be profound, and taking proactive steps to care for your mental health is essential. Here's a comprehensive guide:

1. **Acknowledge Your Emotions:**

- Recognize and validate the range of emotions you may experience, from sadness and frustration to anxiety and grief. Allow yourself the space to feel without judgment.

2. **Open Communication:**

- Maintain open and honest communication with your partner. Share your thoughts, fears, and hopes, fostering a supportive environment for both of you.

3. **Seek Professional Support:**

- Consider therapy or counseling with a mental health professional experienced in fertility issues. This provides a safe space to explore emotions, develop coping strategies, and receive guidance.

4. **Educate Yourself:**

- Gain a thorough understanding of fertility treatments, potential causes of infertility, and available options. Knowledge empowers you to make informed decisions and reduces uncertainty.

5.   **Join Support Groups**:
•   Connect with others experiencing infertility through support groups or online communities. Sharing experiences, insights, and coping strategies can provide a sense of community and reduce feelings of isolation.

6.   **Practice Self-Compassion**:
•   Be kind to yourself. Infertility is challenging, and self-compassion involves treating yourself with the same understanding and support you would offer a friend.

7.   **Establish Healthy Boundaries**:
•   Set boundaries with friends and family regarding discussions about fertility. Decide when and with whom you want to share information, protecting your emotional well-being.

8.   **Mindfulness and Meditation**:
•   Practice mindfulness and meditation to stay present and manage stress. These techniques can help alleviate anxiety and create a sense of calm.

9.   **Prioritize Self-Care**:
•   Incorporate self-care practices into your routine. This may include regular exercise, quality sleep, nutritious meals, and activities that bring you joy.

10.   **Cultivate Hobbies**:
•   Engage in hobbies and activities that bring fulfillment and pleasure. This helps redirect focus and provides a healthy outlet for emotions.

11. **CelebrateNon-Fertility Achievements**:
•   Acknowledge and celebrate personal and professional accomplishments unrelated to fertility. This reinforces a sense of identity beyond the fertility journey.

12.   **Express Yourself Creatively:**
•   Explore creative outlets such as writing, art, or music to express your emotions. Creative expression can be therapeutic and provide a means of processing complex feelings.

13.   **Limit Fertility-Related Stress:**
•   Create a balance by setting aside designated times for fertility-related discussions and allowing yourself breaks from constant focus on the process.

14.   **Connect with Nature**:
•   Spend time outdoors, connecting with nature. Fresh air and natural surroundings can have a positive impact on mental well-being.

15.   **Consider Couples Counseling:**
•   If fertility struggles strain your relationship, consider couples counseling. Professional guidance can help strengthen communication and support each other through the challenges.

16.   **Stay Informed but Take Breaks:**
•   Stay informed about fertility treatments, but allow yourself breaks from constant research. Information overload can contribute to stress.

17. **Explore Spirituality or Mind-Body Practices:**
• Engage in practices that align with your spiritual beliefs or explore mind-body techniques such as yoga or acupuncture, which some find beneficial for mental health during fertility struggles.

Remember, nurturing your mental health is an ongoing process. It's okay to seek help, take breaks, and prioritize your well-being throughout the fertility journey. Taking care of your mental health is a vital aspect of navigating the challenges of infertility with resilience.

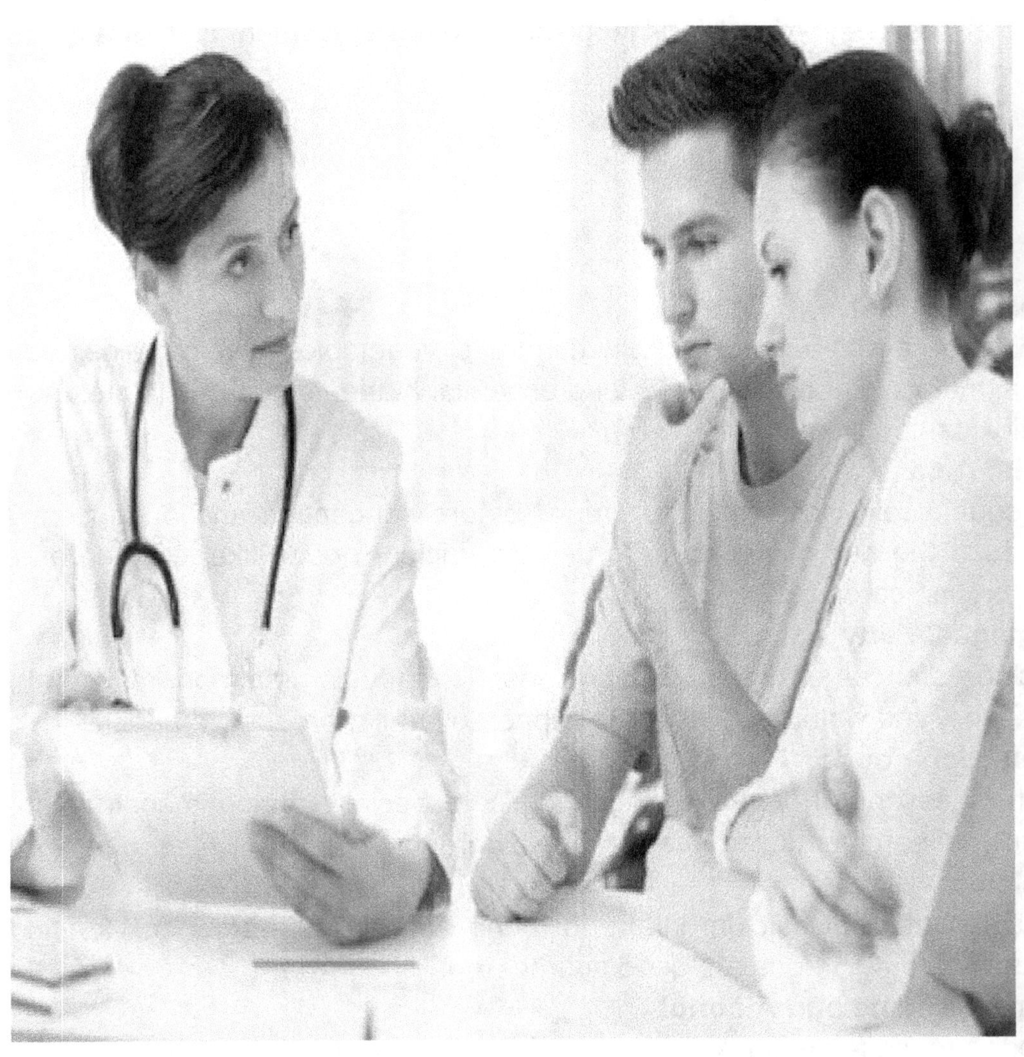

chapter 5. Lifestyle and Holistic Approaches

Nutrition and Wellness for Fertility

Nutrition and wellness play integral roles in reproductive health and fertility. Adopting a healthy lifestyle can positively impact fertility for both men and women. Here's a guide on nutrition and wellness for fertility:

Nutrition for Women

1. **Balanced Diet**
   - Consume a well-balanced diet rich in fruits, vegetables, whole grains, lean proteins, and healthy fats. Ensure you're getting essential nutrients such as folate, iron, calcium, and antioxidants.
2. **Folic Acid**
   - Adequate folic acid intake is crucial before conception and during early pregnancy to reduce the risk of neural tube defects. Include foods like leafy greens, citrus fruits, and fortified cereals.
3. **Omega-3 Fatty Acids**
   - Include sources of omega-3 fatty acids, like fatty fish (salmon, mackerel), flaxseeds, chia seeds, and walnuts. Omega-3s support overall reproductive health.
4. **Iron-Rich Foods**
   - Iron is essential for preventing anemia, especially during menstruation. Good sources include lean meats, legumes, and leafy greens.
5. **Calcium**
   - Ensure sufficient calcium intake for bone health. Dairy products, fortified plant-based milks, and leafy greens are good sources.
6. **Limit Caffeine and Alcohol**
   - Moderate caffeine intake and limit alcohol consumption, as excessive amounts may impact fertility.
7. **Hydration**

• Stay adequately hydrated, as water is essential for overall health and can also support cervical mucus production.

8. **Maintain a Healthy Weight**

• Achieve and maintain a healthy weight. Both underweight and overweight conditions can adversely affect fertility.

9. **Limit Processed Foods**

• Minimize processed foods, as they may contain additives that could impact hormonal balance.

Nutrition for Men

1. **Antioxidant-Rich Diet**

• Consume a diet rich in antioxidants, found in fruits, vegetables, nuts, and whole grains. Antioxidants help protect sperm from oxidative stress.

2. **Zinc**

• Ensure adequate zinc intake, as it is crucial for sperm production. Foods like oysters, beef, and pumpkin seeds are good sources of zinc.

3. **Omega-3 Fatty Acids**

• Include omega-3 fatty acids for sperm health. Fatty fish, flaxseeds, and walnuts are good options.

4. **Vitamins C and E**

• Both vitamins C and E have antioxidant properties that support sperm health. Citrus fruits, berries, almonds, and sunflower seeds are good sources.

5. **Coenzyme Q10 (CoQ10)**

• CoQ10 may help improve sperm motility. Dietary sources include fish, organ meats, and whole grains.

6. **Limit Alcohol and Avoid Excessive Heat**

• Limit alcohol intake, as excessive alcohol can negatively impact sperm quality. Avoid hot tubs or prolonged exposure to excessive heat, which may affect sperm production.

7. **Hydration**

• Men should also stay well-hydrated, as dehydration can affect sperm concentration.

General Wellness Tips

1. **Regular Exercise**:

• Engage in regular, moderate exercise. Physical activity supports overall health and can help manage stress.

2. **Manage Stress**
• Practice stress management techniques such as meditation, yoga, or deep breathing. Chronic stress can impact reproductive hormones.
3. **Adequate Sleep**
• Ensure sufficient and quality sleep. Lack of sleep can disrupt hormonal balance and affect fertility.
4. **Avoid Smoking**
• Quit smoking, as it can harm both male and female fertility.

5. **Regular Check-ups**
• Schedule regular check-ups with healthcare providers to address any underlying health issues that may impact fertility.

Adopting a holistic approach to nutrition and wellness is vital for optimizing fertility. It's recommended to consult with healthcare professionals or nutritionists for personalized advice based on individual health conditions and needs.

Integrative Approaches to Enhance Fertility

integrative approaches, combining conventional and complementary strategies, can be beneficial for enhancing fertility. Here's a concise guide:

Nutrition:
Adopt a well-balanced diet rich in antioxidants, omega-3 fatty acids, and essential nutrients. Consider consulting a nutritionist for personalized guidance.
Acupuncture:
Acupuncture may help improve fertility by promoting blood flow to reproductive organs and reducing stress. Consider sessions with a licensed acupuncturist.
Herbal Supplements:
Some herbs, like chasteberry (Vitex) or maca root, are believed to support hormonal balance. Consult with a healthcare professional before incorporating herbal supplements.
Mind-Body Practices:
Engage in mindfulness, meditation, or yoga to manage stress, which can positively impact reproductive health.
Traditional Chinese Medicine (TCM):
TCM, including acupuncture and herbal medicine, is often used to address imbalances in the body that may affect fertility.
Massage Therapy:

Fertility massage may improve blood circulation to reproductive organs and reduce muscle tension. Seek a therapist with expertise in fertility massage.

Dietary Supplements:

Consider supplements like folic acid, CoQ10, and omega-3 fatty acids. However, consult with a healthcare provider to determine appropriate dosages.

Chiropractic Care:

Some individuals find chiropractic adjustments beneficial for overall wellness and nervous system function, which may indirectly impact fertility.

Biofeedback:

Biofeedback techniques can help individuals manage stress and improve relaxation responses, potentially benefiting fertility.

Aromatherapy:

Some aromatherapy practices, using essential oils like lavender or chamomile, can contribute to relaxation and stress reduction.

Environmental Detoxification:

Minimize exposure to environmental toxins by choosing organic foods, reducing the use of plastics, and considering natural household and personal care products.

Genetic Testing and Counseling:

If recurrent fertility challenges are present, genetic testing and counseling can provide insights into potential genetic factors influencing fertility.

Regular Exercise:

Engage in regular, moderate exercise to support overall health and promote hormonal balance. Avoid excessive or intense exercise that might negatively impact fertility.

Sleep Hygiene:

Prioritize good sleep hygiene. Ensure a consistent sleep schedule and create a conducive sleep environment for quality rest.

Fertility Yoga:

Fertility-specific yoga practices may combine poses and relaxation techniques to support reproductive health and reduce stress.

Remember, integrative approaches should complement, not replace, conventional medical guidance. Always consult with healthcare professionals, including reproductive endocrinologists, before implementing new strategies. The key is to personalize approaches based on individual needs and circumstances.

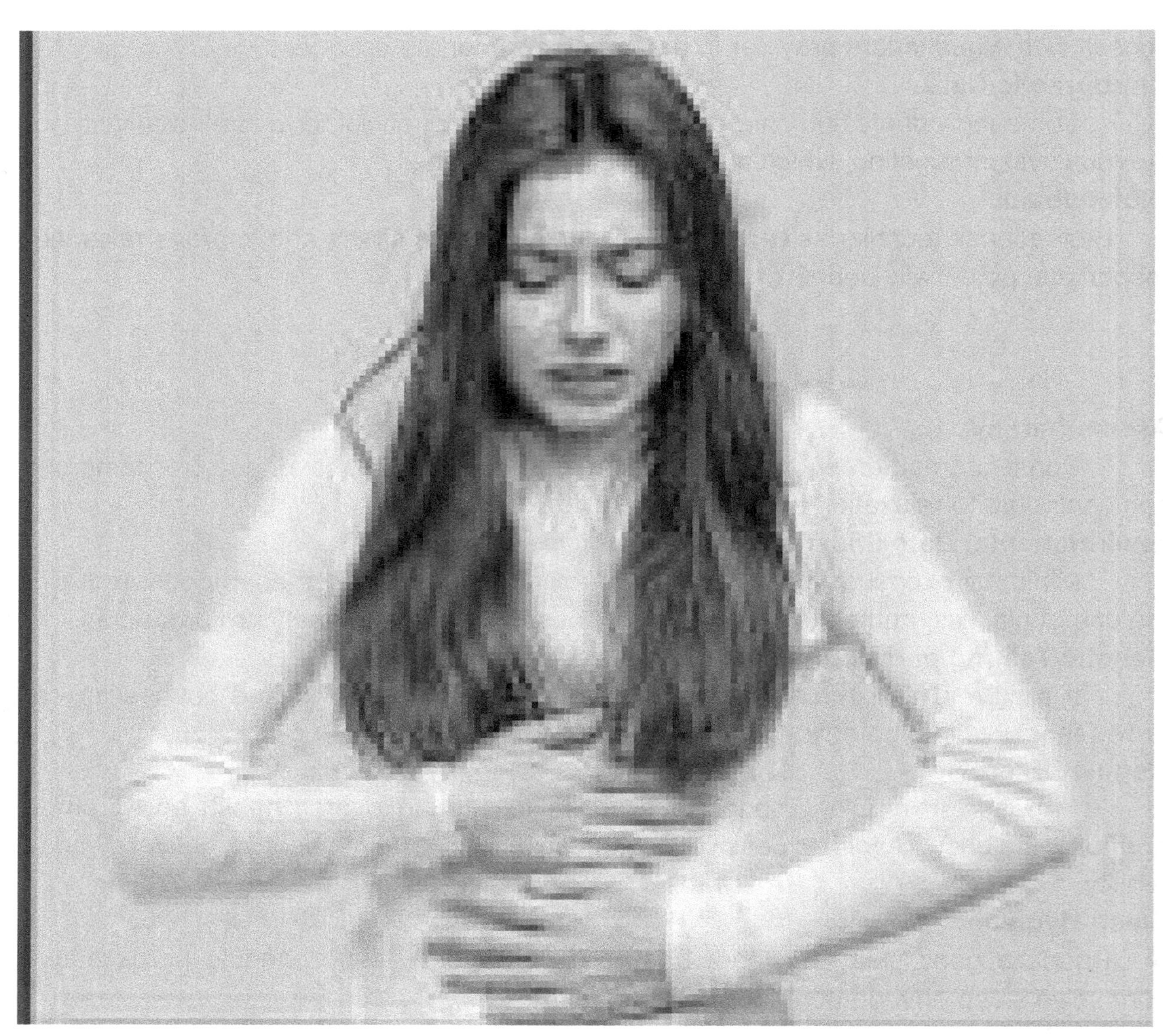

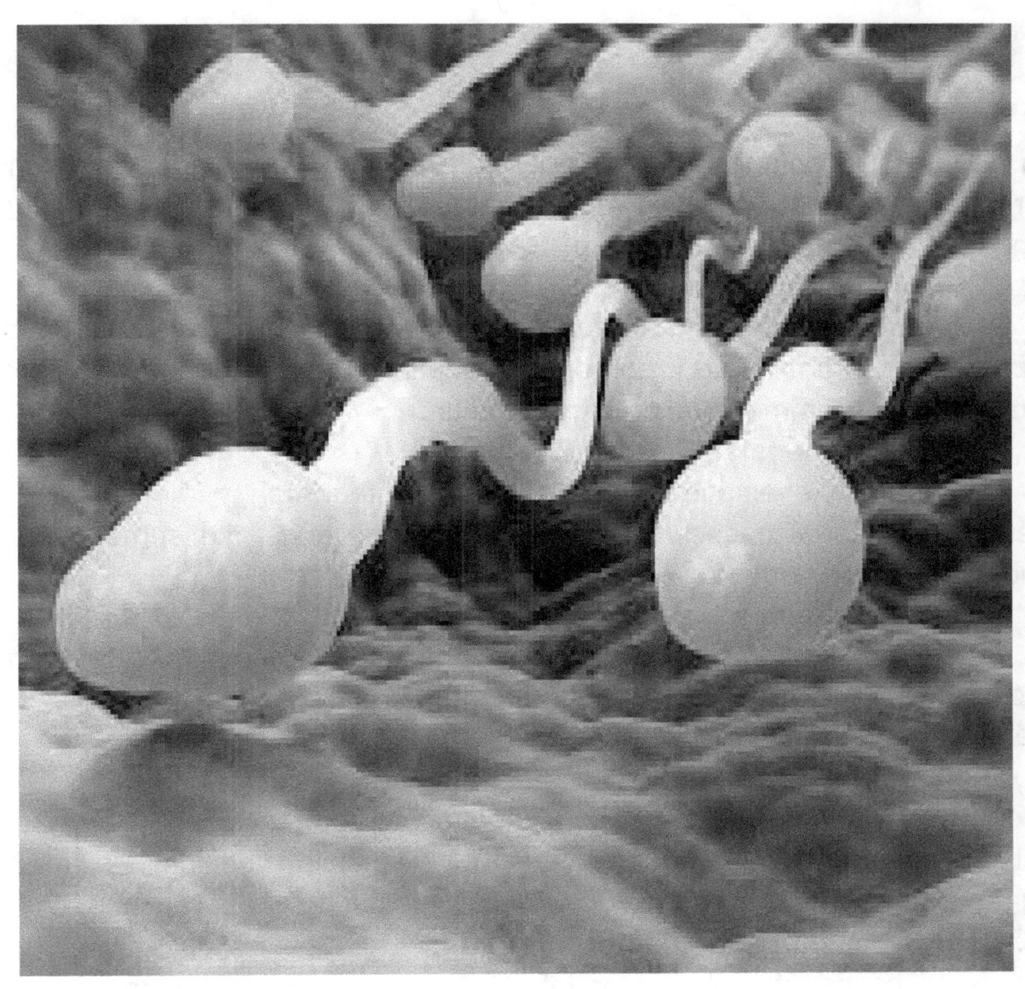

Chapter 6. Support Systems

Seeking Professional Guidance

Seeking professional guidance for infertility is a crucial step toward understanding the underlying causes and exploring appropriate treatments. Here's a guide on the importance of seeking professional help:

1. **Consulting a Reproductive Endocrinologist**:
   - Start by scheduling an appointment with a reproductive endocrinologist, a specialized doctor in fertility and reproductive health. They can conduct comprehensive assessments and recommend tailored treatments.

2. **Comprehensive Fertility Evaluation:**
   - A fertility evaluation typically includes a thorough medical history, physical examinations, hormonal assessments, and diagnostic tests like semen analysis (for men) and ovulation tracking (for women).

3. **Understanding Underlying Causes**:
   - Professionals can identify potential causes of infertility, such as hormonal imbalances, structural issues, or genetic factors. Understanding these factors guides the development of an effective treatment plan.

4. **Tailored Treatment Plans**:
   - Based on the evaluation, healthcare professionals can recommend personalized treatment plans, which may involve lifestyle modifications, medications, assisted reproductive technologies (ART), or a combination of approaches.

5. **Addressing Male Factor Infertility:**
   - In cases of male factor infertility, seeking guidance early allows for a detailed examination of sperm quality and potential causes. Treatments like intracytoplasmic sperm injection (ICSI) or sperm donation may be considered.

6. **Addressing Female Factor Infertility**:
   - For female factor infertility, professionals can explore interventions such as ovulation induction, intrauterine insemination (IUI), or in vitro fertilization (IVF) based on the specific issues identified.

7. **Navigating Unexplained Infertility:**
   - In cases of unexplained infertility, where no clear cause is identified, professionals can guide individuals or couples through a systematic process of exploration and offer evidence-based treatments.

8.   **Psychological Support**:
*   Dealing with infertility can be emotionally challenging. Professionals, including reproductive psychologists or counselors, can provide psychological support and coping strategies throughout the journey.

9.   **Fertility Preservation**:
*   Professionals can discuss options for fertility preservation in cases where medical treatments or conditions may impact future fertility, such as cancer treatments or elective preservation for personal reasons.

10.   **Exploring Alternative Paths:**
*   Healthcare providers can discuss alternative paths to parenthood, including adoption or surrogacy, offering guidance on legal, emotional, and medical aspects.

11.   **Education and Informed Decision-Making:**
*   Seeking professional guidance ensures access to accurate information, allowing individuals and couples to make informed decisions about their fertility journey.

12.   **Monitoring and Adjusting Treatment Plans:**
*   Regular monitoring allows professionals to assess the effectiveness of treatment plans and make necessary adjustments, optimizing the chances of successful conception.

13.   **Addressing Reproductive Health at Every Life Stage:**
*   Fertility specialists can provide guidance on reproductive health at different life stages, from family planning to addressing fertility challenges in advanced maternal age.

14.   **Building a Supportive Network**:
*   Professionals can help individuals or couples build a supportive network, connecting them with resources, support groups, and other individuals facing similar challenges.

15.   **Providing Hope and Encouragement**:
*   Fertility professionals play a crucial role in offering hope, encouragement, and a sense of empowerment throughout the fertility journey.

Seeking professional guidance is a proactive step toward addressing fertility challenges, promoting physical and emotional well-being, and increasing the likelihood of achieving the goal of parenthood.

Relationships Dynamics

Infertility can significantly impact relationship dynamics, testing the resilience and communication between partners. Here's an exploration of the relationship aspects associated with infertility:

Shared Experience

- Facing infertility is a shared experience that can bring couples closer together as they navigate the challenges as a team. Shared understanding fosters a sense of unity.

Communication is Key

- Open and honest communication is crucial. Discussing feelings, fears, and hopes with one another helps prevent emotional distance and strengthens the emotional connection.

Managing Expectations

- Infertility treatments can be emotionally and physically demanding. Managing expectations and understanding the potential ups and downs is important to avoid additional stress on the relationship.

Supporting Each Other

- Providing mutual support is essential. Both partners may experience emotional highs and lows differently, and understanding and supporting each other's coping mechanisms contribute to a supportive environment.

Coping with Grief and Loss

- Experiencing fertility challenges often involves a grieving process for the imagined family trajectory. Supporting each other through the grief and acknowledging the loss is vital for emotional well-being.

Shared Decision-Making

- Decisions about fertility treatments, family planning, and alternative paths to parenthood should be made jointly. Shared decision-making ensures both partners feel heard and respected.

Coping Mechanisms

- Individuals may have different coping mechanisms. While one partner may find solace in sharing feelings, the other might prefer solitary reflection. Respecting these differences is important.

Balancing Personal and Shared Responsibility

- Balancing the emotional and logistical aspects of fertility treatments involves a shared responsibility. Partners may take on different roles, such as scheduling appointments or offering emotional support.

Intimacy Challenges

- The pressure and emotional toll of infertility can affect intimacy. It's important to communicate openly about these challenges, seek professional guidance if needed, and find ways to maintain emotional and physical closeness.

Navigating Social and Family Pressure

- External pressures, comments, or questions from friends and family can add stress. Partners should communicate and establish boundaries together to manage external expectations.

Seeking Professional Support Together

- Engaging in couples counseling or seeking the support of a reproductive psychologist together can provide a safe space for both partners to express concerns and emotions.

Maintaining Emotional Independence

- While supporting each other emotionally, it's also essential for partners to maintain a degree of emotional independence. This allows for personal growth and resilience within the relationship.

Celebrating Milestones Beyond Parenthood

- Couples should continue to celebrate milestones in their relationship beyond the focus on parenthood. This reinforces the importance of the relationship itself.

Addressing Emotional Distance

- If emotional distance emerges, addressing it proactively is crucial. Seeking professional help can be beneficial in navigating these challenges.

Understanding Impact on Identity

- Infertility can impact personal identities as well. Acknowledging and understanding these changes can help partners navigate the complexities of self-identity and identity within the relationship.

Infertility is a shared journey that can either strain or strengthen a relationship. By fostering open communication, mutual support, and shared decision-making, couples can navigate the challenges together, ultimately deepening their connection and resilience.

Relationship Challenges

Infertility can pose significant challenges to relationships, testing the emotional, psychological, and even physical well-being of couples. Here's an exploration of the relationship challenges associated with infertility:

Emotional Strain

- The emotional toll of infertility can lead to heightened stress, anxiety, and feelings of sadness or grief. Couples may struggle with coping mechanisms and emotional regulation.

Communication Breakdowns

- Infertility can strain communication between partners. The sensitive nature of the topic may lead to avoidance or misunderstandings, affecting the overall quality of communication.

Differing Coping Strategies

- Individuals may cope with infertility differently. While one partner may seek solace in sharing emotions, the other may prefer solitude. Understanding and respecting these differences is essential.

Intimacy Issues

- The pressure and emotional strain associated with fertility treatments can impact intimacy. Physical and emotional closeness may decline, leading to feelings of isolation.

Blame and Guilt

- Feelings of blame and guilt can arise, with each partner questioning themselves or each other. Navigating these emotions requires open communication and mutual support.

Social Isolation

- Couples experiencing infertility may withdraw socially, especially if surrounded by friends or family members who have successfully conceived. This isolation can contribute to feelings of loneliness.

Loss of Spontaneity

- Fertility treatments often involve strict schedules and routines. This loss of spontaneity can affect the natural flow of the relationship, leading to additional stress.

Financial Strain

- Fertility treatments can be financially burdensome. Disagreements over the cost, the extent of treatments, or financial priorities can create tension within the relationship.

Dealing with External Pressures

- Comments or inquiries from well-meaning friends and family can exacerbate stress. Couples may feel pressure to provide updates or explanations, leading to additional emotional strain.

Impact on Self-Esteem

- Infertility challenges can impact self-esteem and self-worth. Individuals may feel inadequate, leading to internal struggles that spill over into the relationship.

Loss of Control

- The unpredictability of fertility treatments and outcomes can evoke a sense of loss of control. Couples may grapple with uncertainty, further straining their emotional resilience.

Coping with Treatment Failures

- Experiencing failed fertility treatments can be devastating. Couples must navigate grief and disappointment together, seeking support when needed.

Balancing Work and Treatment

- The demands of fertility treatments may conflict with work responsibilities, causing additional stress. Couples need to find a balance that works for both partners.

Impact on Sexual Intimacy

- The medicalized nature of fertility treatments can alter the nature of sexual intimacy. Partners may struggle with viewing sex as a means to an end rather than a spontaneous, intimate connection.

Decision-Making Fatigue

- The constant decision-making involved in fertility treatments can lead to decision fatigue,

In summary, relationship challenges are an inevitable part of the human experience. Whether stemming from external pressures, communication breakdowns, or life transitions, these challenges provide opportunities for growth, understanding, and resilience. By fostering open communication, empathy, and a willingness to navigate difficulties together, couples can transform challenges into catalysts for stronger, more resilient relationships. Embracing these challenges as shared experiences can ultimately lead to deeper connections and a more profound understanding of one another.

Chapter 7. Decision-Making

Considering Alternative Paths to Parenthood

Considering alternative paths to parenthood is an important and personal decision for individuals or couples facing infertility. Exploring various options requires careful consideration and understanding. Here's a comprehensive guide:

Acceptance and Open Communication

- Acknowledge and accept the reality of infertility. Open communication between partners is crucial to understanding each other's feelings and exploring alternative paths together.

Educate Yourself

- Research and gather information about different paths to parenthood. Understand the processes, legal aspects, and emotional implications associated with adoption, surrogacy, and other options.

Adoption

- Explore domestic and international adoption options. Consider factors such as adoption agencies, legal requirements, and the emotional aspects of welcoming a child into your family who may not share a biological connection.

Foster Care

- Investigate foster care as a potential path. This involves providing a temporary home for children in need. Understand the legal and emotional aspects involved in fostering and potential avenues for adoption through foster care.

Surrogacy

- Consider gestational surrogacy, where a woman carries a child to term for another individual or couple. Understand the legal, financial, and ethical considerations, and choose a reputable surrogacy agency if pursuing this path.

Egg or Sperm Donation

- Explore using donor eggs or sperm to achieve pregnancy through in vitro fertilization (IVF). Understand the ethical and legal implications, as well as the emotional aspects involved in using a donor's genetic material.

Legal Considerations

- Familiarize yourself with the legal aspects of alternative paths to parenthood, including adoption laws, surrogacy regulations, and any requirements associated with assisted reproductive technologies.

Financial Planning

- Assess the financial implications of different paths. Adoption, surrogacy, and assisted reproductive technologies can involve significant costs. Budgeting and financial planning are crucial considerations.

Emotional Preparedness

- Reflect on your emotional readiness for alternative paths. Understand that each option comes with its own set of challenges and joys. Counseling or support groups can provide valuable insights and emotional support.

Cultural and Religious Considerations

- Consider cultural and religious factors that may influence your decisions. Some cultures or religious beliefs may impact the acceptance of certain alternative paths to parenthood.

Family and Social Support

- Assess the level of support from family and friends. Having a supportive network can positively impact the experience of exploring alternative paths to parenthood.

Personal Values and Beliefs

- Reflect on your personal values and beliefs surrounding family, parenthood, and the importance of biological connections. This introspection can guide decision-making.

13. **Timing and Patience:**

- Understand that each alternative path may involve varying timelines. Be patient and realistic about the time commitment required for the chosen path.

Legal Consultation

- Seek legal advice to understand the legal intricacies associated with your chosen alternative path. This is especially important in international adoption, surrogacy, and assisted reproductive technologies.

Continuous Reevaluation

- Recognize that feelings and circumstances may change over time. Continuously reevaluate your choices and be open to adjusting your path based on evolving circumstances or preferences.

Community and Peer Support

- Connect with communities or support groups that focus on the alternative path you are considering. Learning from others who have gone through similar experiences can be valuable.

Professional Guidance

- Consult with professionals such as adoption agencies, fertility specialists, or legal experts. Their expertise can provide guidance and clarity as you navigate alternative paths to parenthood.

Ultimately, the decision to pursue alternative paths to parenthood is deeply personal. Taking the time to explore, understand, and communicate openly with your partner ensures that you make choices aligned with your values, preferences, and the

Family Planning and Decision Points

Family planning in the context of infertility involves navigating a complex journey with various decision points. Here's a comprehensive guide to help individuals or couples facing infertility make informed choices:

Initial Consultation

- Schedule an initial consultation with a reproductive endocrinologist or fertility specialist. This step involves a comprehensive evaluation of both partners to identify potential causes of infertility.

Understanding Diagnosis

- Gain a thorough understanding of the diagnosis. Identify whether the infertility is due to male factors, female factors, a combination of both, or unexplained causes.

Lifestyle Modifications

- Implement lifestyle changes to optimize fertility. This may include maintaining a healthy weight, adopting a balanced diet, managing stress, and avoiding substances like tobacco and excessive alcohol.

Treatment Options

- Discuss and understand the range of fertility treatments available. This may include ovulation induction, intrauterine insemination (IUI), and in vitro fertilization (IVF). Explore the potential risks, success rates, and financial implications of each.

Financial Planning

- Assess the financial implications of fertility treatments. Consider insurance coverage, out-of-pocket costs, and potential expenses associated with multiple treatment cycles.

Emotional Readiness

- Evaluate emotional readiness for fertility treatments. Recognize that the process may involve emotional highs and lows, and consider seeking support from mental health professionals or support groups.

Natural Conception vs. Assisted Reproductive Technologies (ART)

- Decide whether to pursue natural conception, assisted reproductive technologies, or a combination of both. Consider personal preferences, timeline, and the emotional and financial investment associated with each option.

Timelines and Patience

- Set realistic timelines for family planning. Understand that fertility treatments may take time, and multiple cycles might be necessary. Patience and perseverance are key.

Medication Options

- If medications are recommended, understand the purpose, potential side effects, and administration methods. Discuss any concerns with your healthcare provider.

Intrauterine Insemination (IUI)

- Explore the option of IUI. Understand the process, success rates, and conditions under which it might be recommended.

In Vitro Fertilization (IVF)

- Consider IVF as a potential option. Understand the steps involved, success rates, and potential challenges. Discuss any ethical or moral considerations related to IVF.

Genetic Testing

- Discuss the option of genetic testing. Understand the purpose, types of testing available, and how results might influence treatment decisions.

Third-Party Reproduction

- Explore third-party reproduction options, such as egg or sperm donation or using a gestational carrier. Understand the legal, ethical, and emotional aspects associated with these options.

Adoption and Surrogacy

- If fertility treatments are not successful or are not the preferred path, explore adoption or surrogacy. Understand the legal and emotional considerations associated with each option.

Counseling and Support

- Engage in counseling or support groups to navigate the emotional aspects of family planning. Seeking professional guidance can provide coping strategies and emotional support.

Legal Considerations

- Understand the legal aspects associated with different family planning options, especially when considering surrogacy or adoption. Seek legal advice to ensure a clear understanding of your rights and responsibilities.

Reevaluation and Flexibility

- Continuously reevaluate family planning decisions. Be flexible and open to adjusting the plan based on evolving circumstances, treatment outcomes, or personal preferences.

Communication with Partner

- Maintain open and honest communication with your partner throughout the process. Share feelings, concerns, and hopes to ensure you are on the same page.

Child-Free Living

- Consider and discuss the possibility of living child-free. Acknowledge that family planning can take unexpected turns, and being open to this option can reduce stress.

Reflection on Values and Priorities

- Reflect on personal values, priorities, and the vision for family life. Family planning decisions should align with your beliefs and long-term goals.

Navigating family planning decisions in the context of infertility involves careful consideration, collaboration with healthcare professionals, and open communication within the partnership. It's a unique journey for each individual or couple, and finding a path that aligns with personal values and goals is paramount.

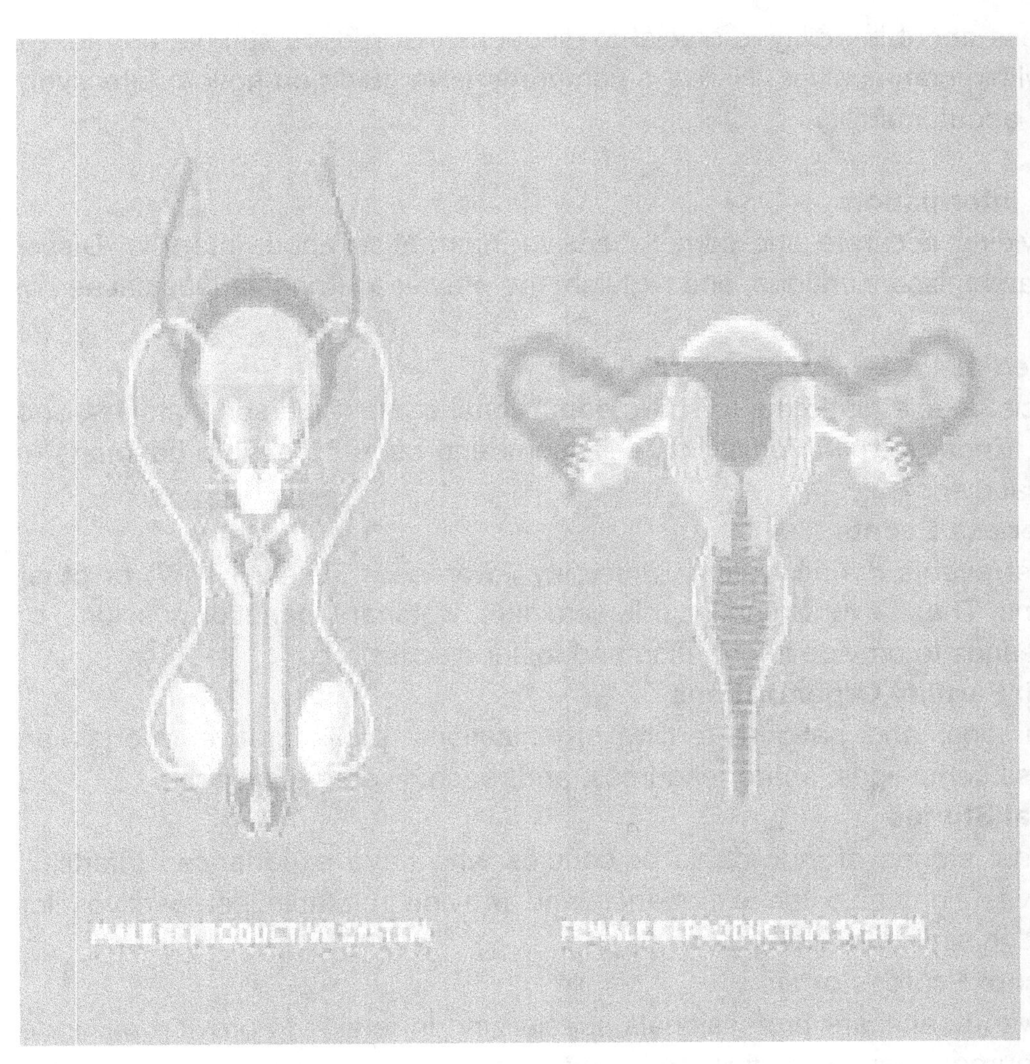

MALE REPRODUCTIVE SYSTEM
FEMALE REPRODUCTIVE SYSTEM

Chapter 8. Advocacy and Education

Raising Awareness about Infertility

Raising awareness about infertility is crucial to dispel myths, reduce stigma, and foster understanding within communities. Here's a comprehensive guide on how to effectively raise awareness about infertility:

***Education and Information**
  - Start by providing accurate and comprehensive information about infertility. Dispel common myths and misconceptions, and highlight the prevalence and various causes of infertility.

Utilize Social Media
  - Leverage social media platforms to share educational content, personal stories, and relevant articles. Engage with infertility organizations and use appropriate hashtags to reach a broader audience.

Organize Awareness Events
  - Plan and host events during National Infertility Awareness Week (NIAW) or other relevant occasions. These events can include seminars, webinars, panel discussions, or community gatherings to provide information and foster discussions.

Collaborate with Fertility Organizations
  - Partner with local and national fertility organizations. Collaborative efforts can amplify awareness campaigns, share resources, and reach diverse audiences.

Feature Personal Stories
  - Share personal stories of individuals or couples who have experienced infertility. Personal narratives humanize the experience and provide relatable perspectives for those going through similar challenges.

Engage Healthcare Professionals
  - Collaborate with healthcare professionals specializing in fertility to provide accurate information. Encourage them to participate in awareness campaigns or share resources in their practices.

School and Workplace Initiatives
  - Implement educational initiatives in schools and workplaces. Work with educators and employers to incorporate discussions about infertility, family planning, and support systems.

Create Infertility Awareness Materials
  - Develop informative materials such as brochures, posters, and online resources. Distribute these materials in healthcare settings, community centers, and public spaces.

Lobby for Legislative Support

- Advocate for policies that support individuals and couples dealing with infertility. Raise awareness about the need for insurance coverage, workplace accommodations, and fertility treatment accessibility.

Utilize Celebrity Endorsement

- Collaborate with celebrities or influencers who are open about their fertility journeys. Their endorsement can significantly increase the reach and impact of awareness campaigns.

Engage Religious and Cultural Communities

- Approach religious and cultural leaders to discuss infertility within their communities. Addressing the topic in religious or cultural contexts can help reduce stigma and foster support.

Online Webinars and Podcasts

- Host webinars and podcasts featuring experts, patients, and advocates. These digital platforms provide accessible and interactive spaces for education and discussion.

Participate in Health Fairs

- Set up information booths at health fairs or community events. Distribute materials, answer questions, and engage with the public to raise awareness.

Media Partnerships

- Collaborate with media outlets to share stories and educational content. Feature articles, interviews, or documentaries that shed light on the diverse aspects of infertility.

Workplace Awareness Programs

- Encourage workplaces to implement infertility awareness programs. This can include seminars, counseling services, and policies that support employees dealing with fertility challenges.

Incorporate Infertility in Sex Education

- Advocate for the inclusion of infertility awareness in sex education programs. This can help young individuals understand the importance of reproductive health and family planning.

International Collaboration

- Connect with international organizations and participate in global awareness campaigns. Understanding infertility from a global perspective can broaden the conversation and address cultural nuances.

Provide Resources for Support

- Share information about support groups, counseling services, and mental health resources for individuals and couples dealing with infertility.

Continuous Engagement

- Keep the momentum going beyond specific awareness periods. Continuous engagement ensures that infertility remains part of ongoing conversations and efforts.

Monitor and Evaluate Impact
   - Regularly assess the impact of awareness campaigns. Collect feedback, analyze engagement metrics, and adjust strategies accordingly for greater effectiveness.

Raising awareness about infertility is an ongoing effort that requires collaboration, empathy, and a commitment to dispelling stigma. By combining education, personal stories, and community engagement, you can contribute to fostering a more informed and supportive environment for those navigating the challenges of infertility.

Accessing Educational Resources

To access educational resources on infertility, follow these steps:

Online Research
   Begin by conducting online research on reputable websites such as the American Society for Reproductive Medicine (ASRM), Resolve: The National Infertility Association, and the Mayo Clinic. These sources offer a wealth of information on infertility causes, treatments, and support.

Medical Journals and Publications
   Explore medical journals and publications dedicated to reproductive health. Journals like Fertility and Sterility or Human Reproduction often provide in-depth research articles and studies. PubMed is a valuable database for accessing scientific literature.

Bookstores and Libraries
   Visit local bookstores or libraries to find books on infertility written by experts in the field. Titles like "Taking Charge of Your Fertility" by Toni Weschler or "The Infertility Cure" by Randine Lewis can offer insightful perspectives.

Online Courses and Webinars
   Enroll in online courses or attend webinars hosted by fertility experts and organizations. Platforms like Coursera, Udemy, or specialized fertility education websites may offer courses on understanding infertility, treatment options, and emotional well-being.

Fertility Clinics and Specialists
   Consult fertility clinics and specialists for personalized guidance. Many clinics host informational sessions or provide educational materials. Schedule appointments to discuss your specific situation and gather resources tailored to your needs.

Support Groups

Join infertility support groups, either in person or online. Platforms like RESOLVE or BabyCenter host forums where individuals share experiences, information, and resources. Connecting with others going through similar challenges can be invaluable.

Educational Events and Conferences

Attend fertility-related events and conferences. These gatherings often feature expert speakers, panel discussions, and workshops covering various aspects of infertility. Check the schedules of organizations like ASRM for upcoming events.

Social Media and Podcasts

Follow reputable fertility experts, organizations, and podcasts on social media platforms. Many experts share informative content, research updates, and resources. Podcasts like "The Fertility Podcast" or "Beat Infertility" can provide valuable insights.

Government Health Agencies

Explore resources provided by government health agencies. In the United States, the Centers for Disease Control and Prevention (CDC) and the National Institute of Child Health and Human Development (NICHD) offer information on infertility and reproductive health.

Ask Your Healthcare Provider

Consult with your healthcare provider for recommended resources. They can provide pamphlets, brochures, and direct you to reliable sources based on your specific situation.

Remember to critically evaluate the credibility of the sources you consult and consult with healthcare professionals for personalized advice. Infertility can be complex, and seeking information from multiple reputable sources is crucial.

Chapter 9. Conclusion

Embracing Hope and Resilience

Embracing hope and resilience while navigating infertility can be challenging, but it's a crucial aspect of maintaining emotional well-being. Here are some strategies to help you foster hope and resilience:

1. Educate Yourself

Gain a deep understanding of infertility, its causes, and available treatments. Knowledge can empower you to make informed decisions and better cope with the emotional rollercoaster.

2. Set Realistic Goals

Establish achievable goals on your fertility journey. This might involve setting realistic expectations for treatments, acknowledging potential setbacks, and celebrating small victories along the way.

3. Create a Support System

Build a strong support network that includes your partner, family, friends, and support groups. Sharing your feelings and experiences with others who understand can provide comfort and encouragement.

4. Seek Professional Support

Consult with mental health professionals, such as therapists or counselors, specializing in fertility-related issues. They can offer coping strategies, emotional support, and a safe space to express your feelings.

5. Practice Self-Care

Prioritize self-care to nurture your mental and emotional well-being. Engage in activities that bring you joy, relaxation, and a sense of fulfillment. This might include exercise, meditation, or pursuing hobbies.

6. Mindfulness and Meditation

Incorporate mindfulness and meditation into your daily routine. These practices can help manage stress, reduce anxiety, and enhance your ability to stay present in the moment.

7. Celebrate Milestones

Acknowledge and celebrate milestones, whether they're related to your fertility journey or personal achievements. Recognizing progress, no matter how small, can contribute to a positive mindset.

8. Maintain Open Communication

Foster open communication with your partner throughout the journey. Share your thoughts, fears, and hopes, and encourage your partner to do the same. Strong communication can strengthen your relationship.

9. Set Boundaries

Establish boundaries to protect your emotional well-being. This may involve limiting conversations about fertility with certain individuals, taking breaks from fertility-related activities, or avoiding triggers that exacerbate stress.

10. Explore Alternative Paths

Be open to exploring alternative family-building paths, such as adoption or surrogacy. Flexibility in your family-building plan can alleviate the pressure and open new doors to parenthood.

11. Cultivate Positivity

Surround yourself with positive influences, whether through inspirational quotes, affirmations, or engaging in activities that uplift your spirits. Cultivating a positive mindset can contribute to resilience.

12. Set Realistic Timelines

Understand that fertility journeys can be unpredictable. While it's essential to have a plan, be flexible with timelines and be patient with the process.

Embracing hope and resilience involves a combination of self-care, support, and adapting to the unpredictability of the fertility journey. Remember that it's okay to seek help and take breaks when needed, and focus on building a foundation of emotional strength for the road ahead.

Moving Forward with Empowerment and Understanding

Moving forward with empowerment and understanding in the face of infertility requires a holistic approach. Here's a comprehensive guide to help you navigate this journey:

Acknowledge Emotions

Start by acknowledging and understanding your emotions. Infertility can evoke a range of feelings, from frustration to sadness. Allow yourself to experience and express these emotions without judgment.

Educate Yourself

Equip yourself with knowledge about infertility causes, treatments, and options. Understanding the medical aspects can empower you to make informed decisions and actively participate in your fertility journey.

Set Realistic Expectations

Establish realistic expectations for the road ahead. Recognize that fertility treatments may involve ups and downs, and outcomes can vary. Setting realistic expectations can help manage stress and disappointment.

Advocate for Yourself

Be an active advocate for your fertility journey. Ask questions, seek second opinions, and communicate openly with your healthcare team. Your voice is essential in making decisions that align with your values and preferences.

Counseling and Support Services

Consider seeking counseling or support services. Professional therapists and support groups can provide emotional support, coping strategies, and a safe space to share experiences with others facing similar challenges.

Include Your Partner

Involve your partner in the decision-making process. Foster open communication, and ensure that both partners feel heard and understood. Facing infertility together strengthens the bond between partners.

Explore Holistic Approaches

Explore holistic approaches to complement medical treatments. Practices such as acupuncture, yoga, and dietary changes may positively impact overall well-being and fertility.

Embrace Alternative Paths

Be open to alternative family-building paths. Adoption, surrogacy, or other options may offer new possibilities and allow you to build a family in ways you may not have initially considered.

Prioritize Self-Care

Prioritize self-care to nurture your physical and mental well-being. Ensure you get enough rest, engage in activities you enjoy, and practice mindfulness to reduce stress.

Advocate for Fertility Coverage

Advocate for increased awareness and insurance coverage for fertility treatments. Participate in advocacy efforts to promote accessibility and affordability of fertility care.

Celebrate Milestones

Celebrate both personal and fertility-related milestones. This might include completing a treatment cycle, reaching emotional breakthroughs, or achieving personal goals unrelated to fertility.

Plan for the Future

Develop a flexible plan for the future that includes family-building goals and alternative paths. Having a plan provides a sense of direction while allowing room for adaptation as circumstances evolve.

Connect with the Community

Engage with the infertility community through online forums, social media groups, or local support networks. Sharing experiences and insights with others who understand can provide a sense of belonging and encouragement.

Stay Informed on Research

Keep abreast of advancements in fertility research and technologies. Staying informed may open up new possibilities and treatment options.Empowering yourself and moving forward with understanding in the realm of infertility involves a combination of education, emotional support, and proactive decision-making. By taking a holistic approach and embracing various resources, you can navigate this journey with resilience and empowerment.

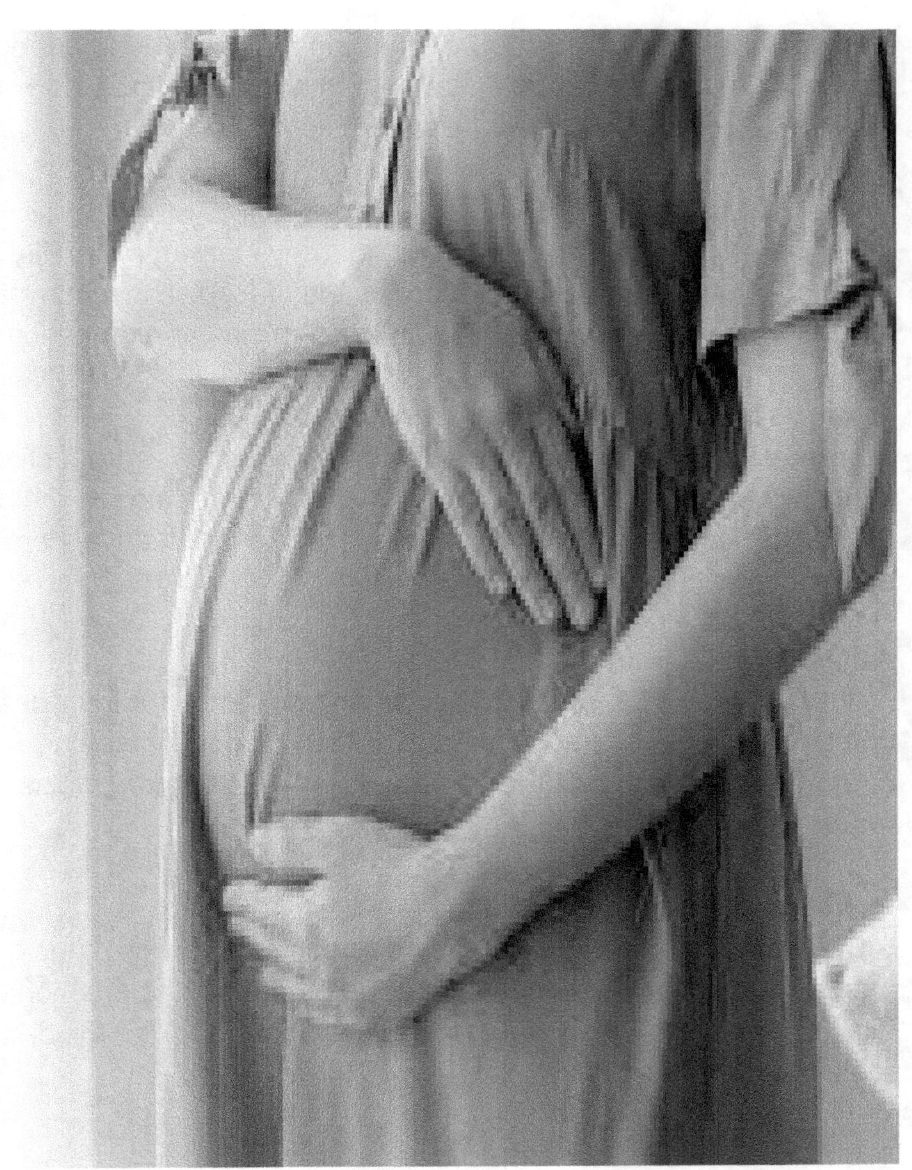

About author

Authors who write on infertility often bring a unique blend of personal experience, professional expertise, and empathy to their work. Here's an overview of what you might find in the works of authors who tackle the topic:

Personal Narratives

Many authors share their personal journeys through infertility, offering a glimpse into the emotional and physical challenges they faced. These narratives can provide comfort and understanding to readers going through similar experiences.

Expertise in Reproductive Health

Some authors bring a professional background in reproductive health, medicine, or psychology to their writing. Their works may delve into the medical aspects of infertility, discussing causes, treatment options, and the latest advancements in reproductive technologies.

Advice and Guidance

Authors often offer practical advice and guidance for individuals navigating the complexities of infertility. This may include insights on coping with emotional stress, communicating with healthcare professionals, or making decisions about fertility treatments.

Holistic Approaches

Certain authors explore holistic approaches to fertility, considering not only the medical aspect but also the importance of mental and emotional well-being. They may discuss lifestyle changes, alternative therapies, and the mind-body connection in relation to fertility.

Advocacy and Awareness

Many authors use their platform to advocate for increased awareness and understanding of infertility. They may address societal perceptions, advocate for policy changes, and work to reduce the stigma associated with fertility challenges.

Educational Resources

Authors often compile comprehensive educational resources on infertility, providing readers with a one-stop reference for information on causes, treatments, and support options. These resources may be accessible to both individuals experiencing infertility and healthcare professionals.

Support and Encouragement

Writing on infertility often includes a strong element of support and encouragement. Authors may share stories of resilience, triumph over adversity, and the importance of maintaining hope throughout the journey.

Parenting After Infertility

Some authors extend their focus to the unique experiences of parenting after infertility. They may address the emotional complexities, joys, and challenges of building a family after fertility struggles.

*Fictional Representations

In addition to non-fiction works, some authors incorporate infertility themes into fiction. This allows for a creative exploration of the emotional nuances surrounding infertility through characters and narratives.

Community Building

Authors may actively engage with their readers and the infertility community through social media, blogs, or other platforms. This community building fosters a sense of connection and solidarity among individuals facing similar challenges.

Examples of authors in this field include Randine Lewis, who wrote "The Infertility Cure," and Julia Indichova, author of "Inconceivable." These authors and others contribute significantly to the wealth of resources available for those seeking information, support, and understanding on the topic of infertility.

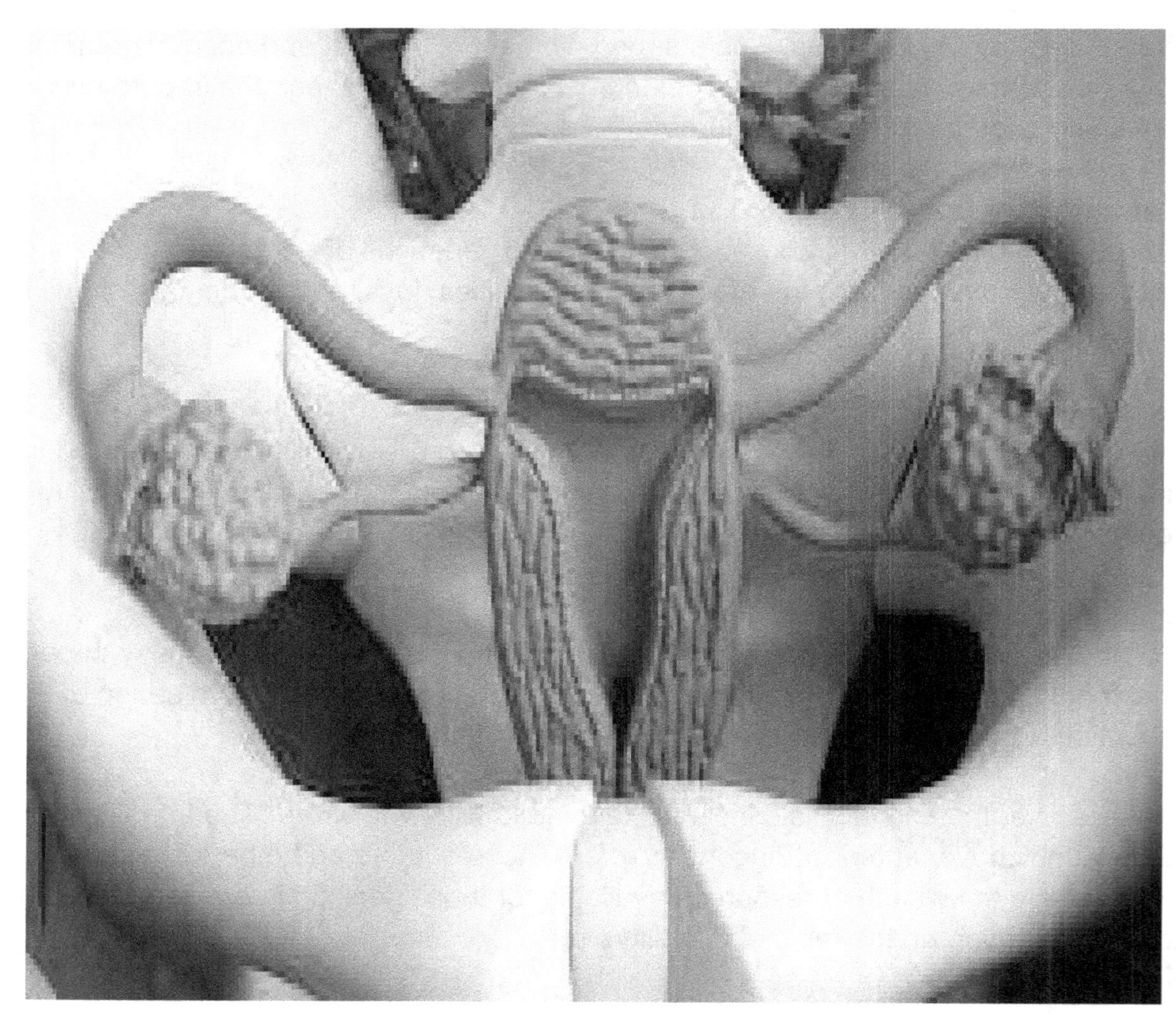

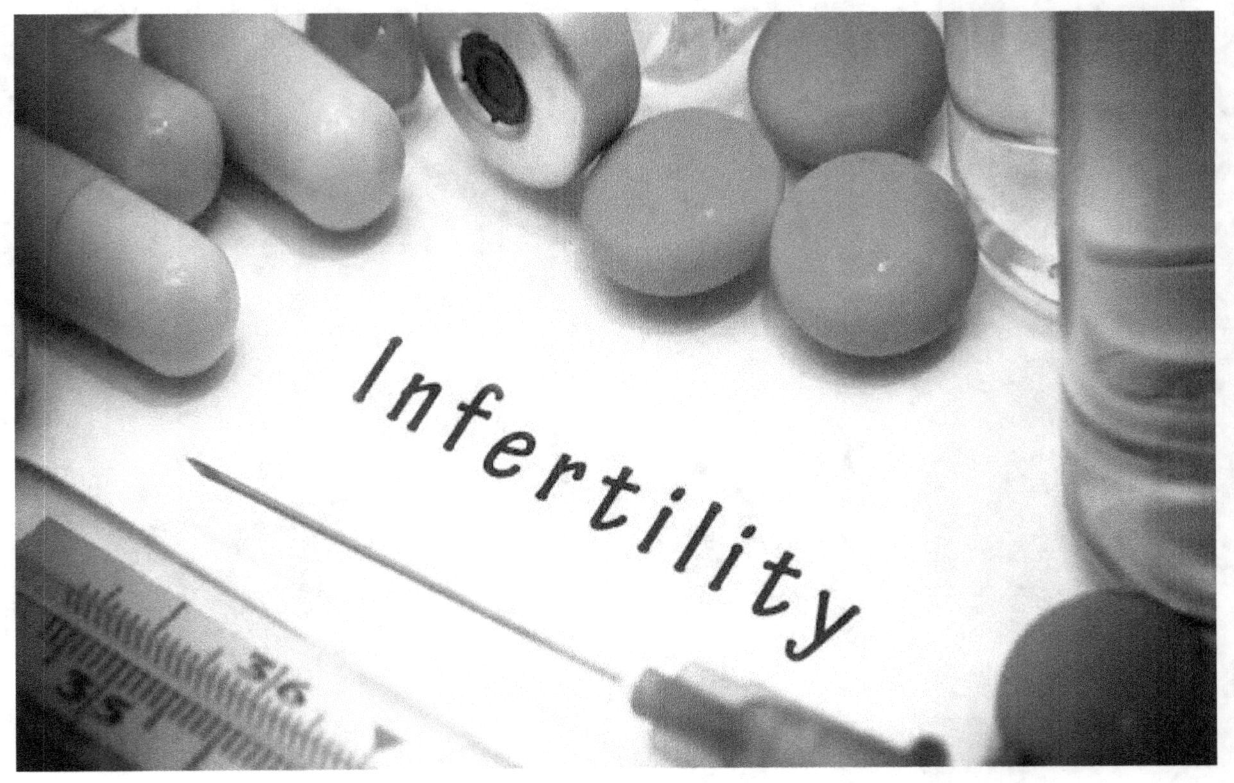
Infertility

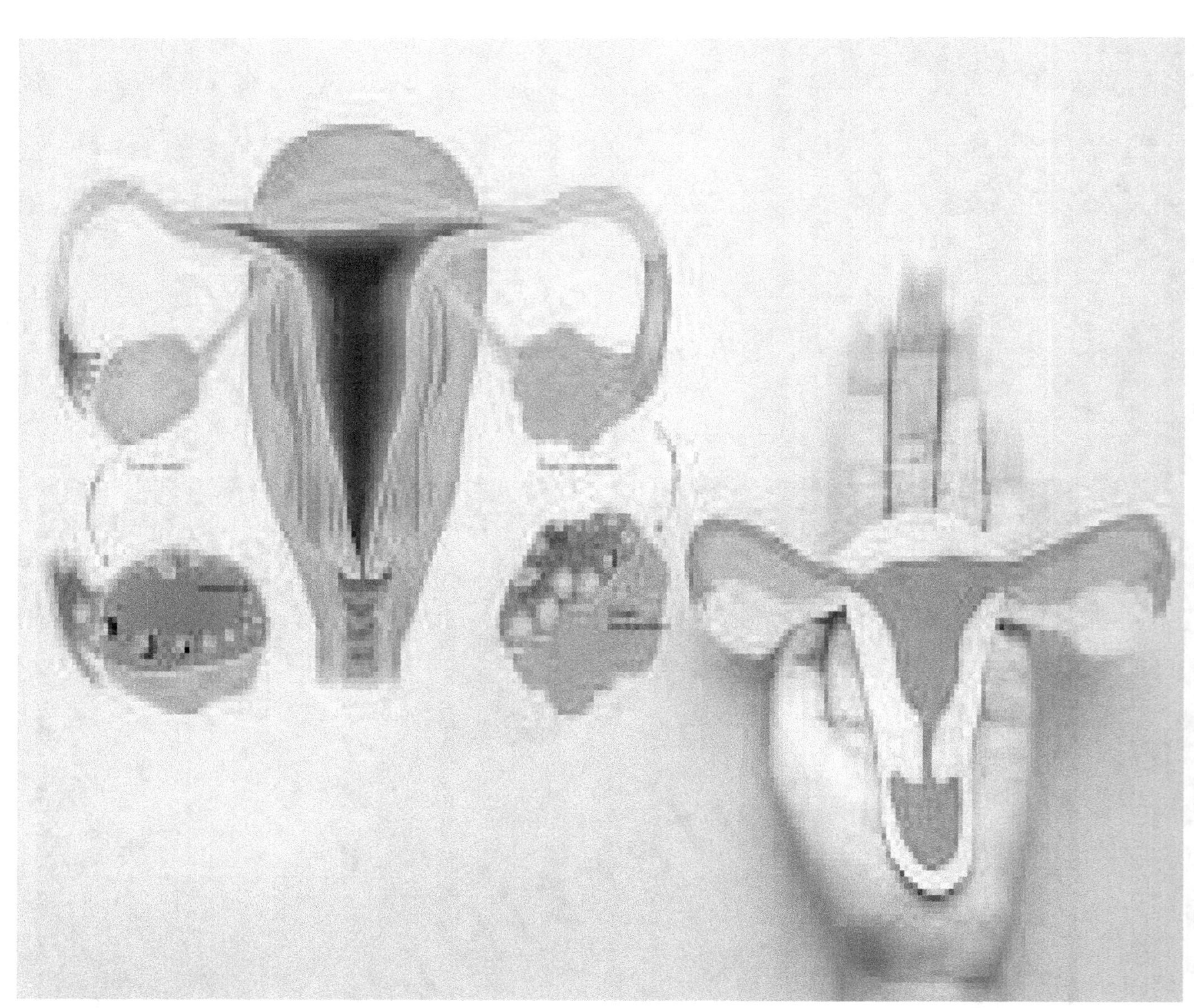

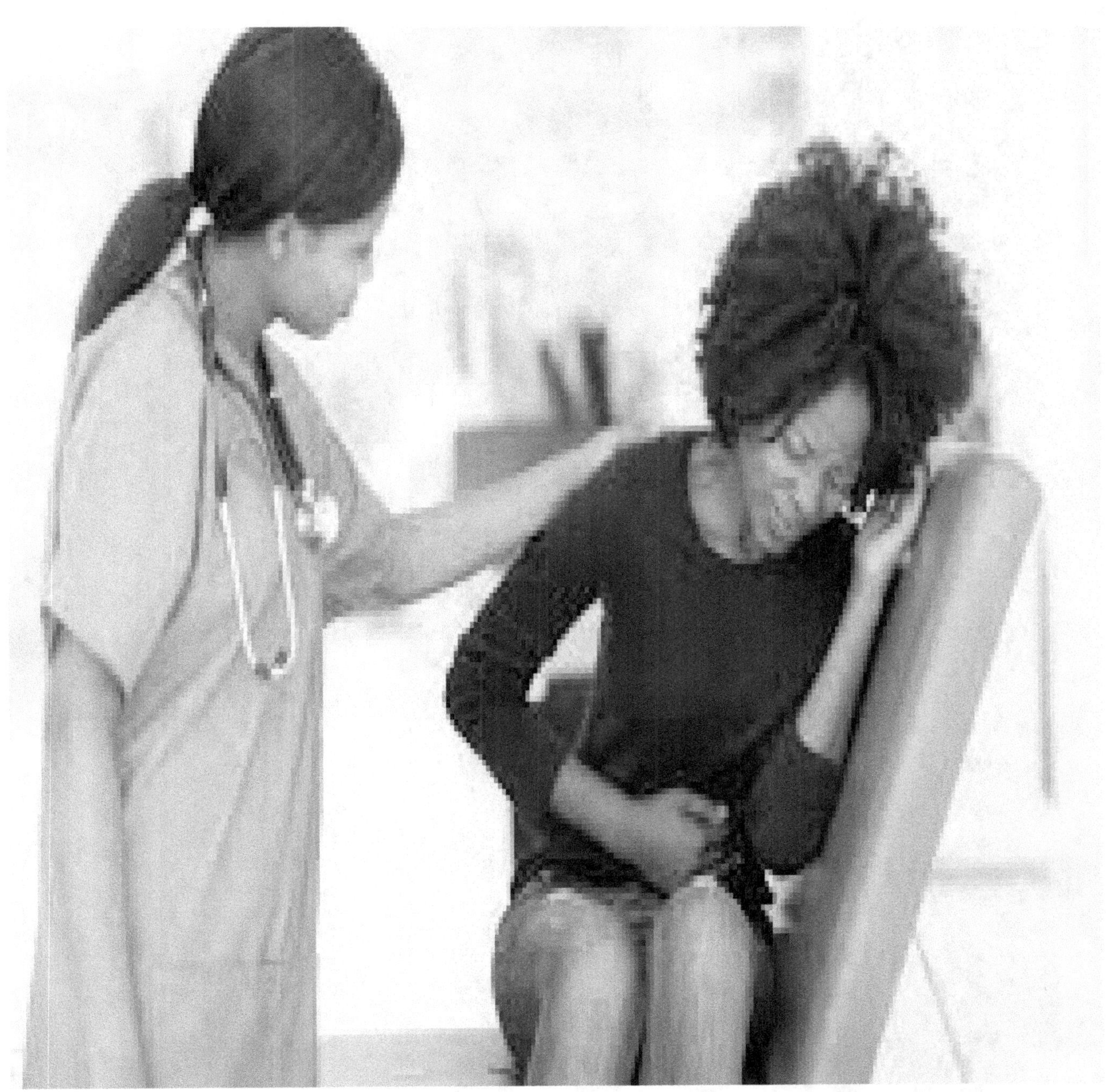

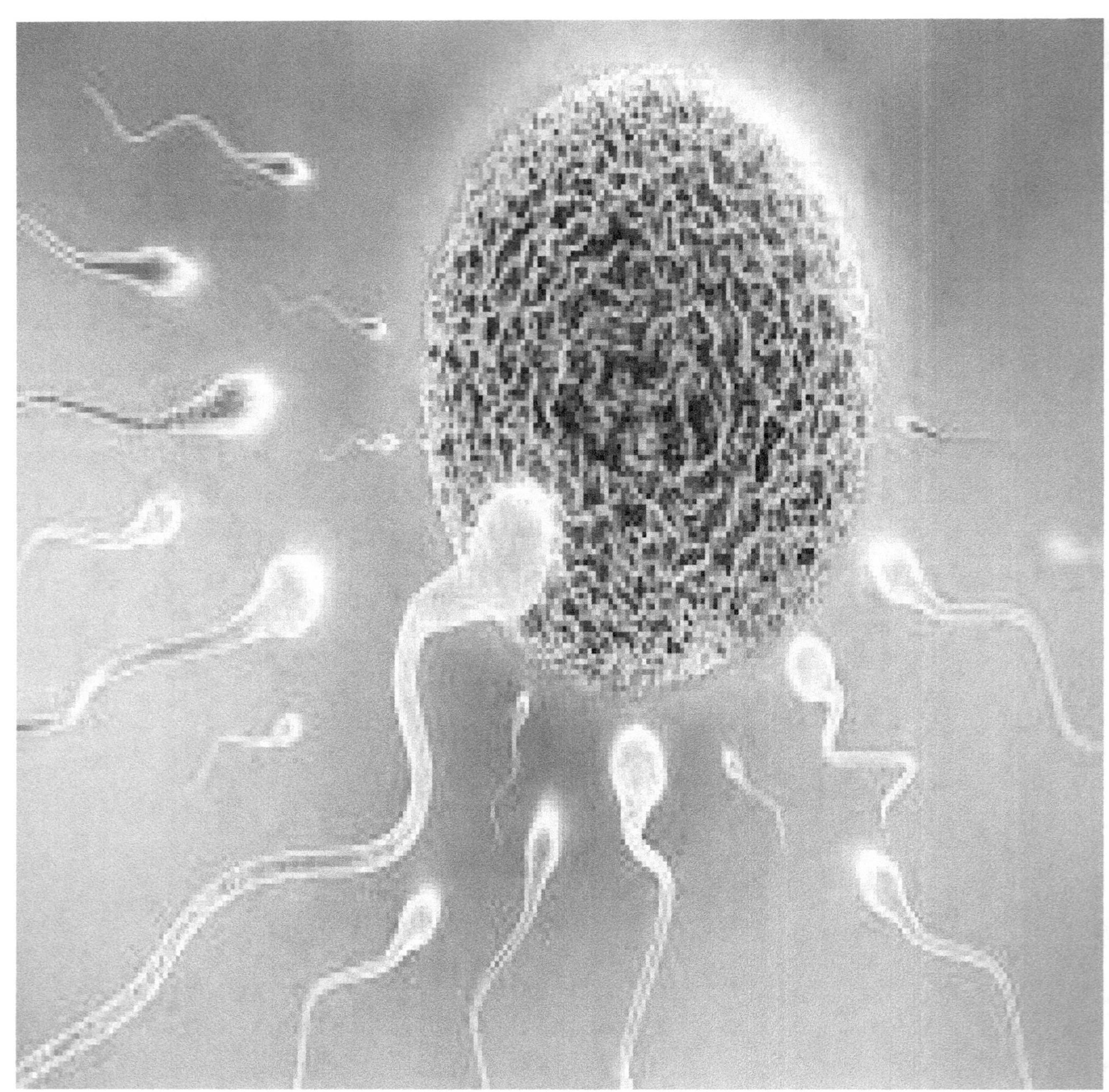

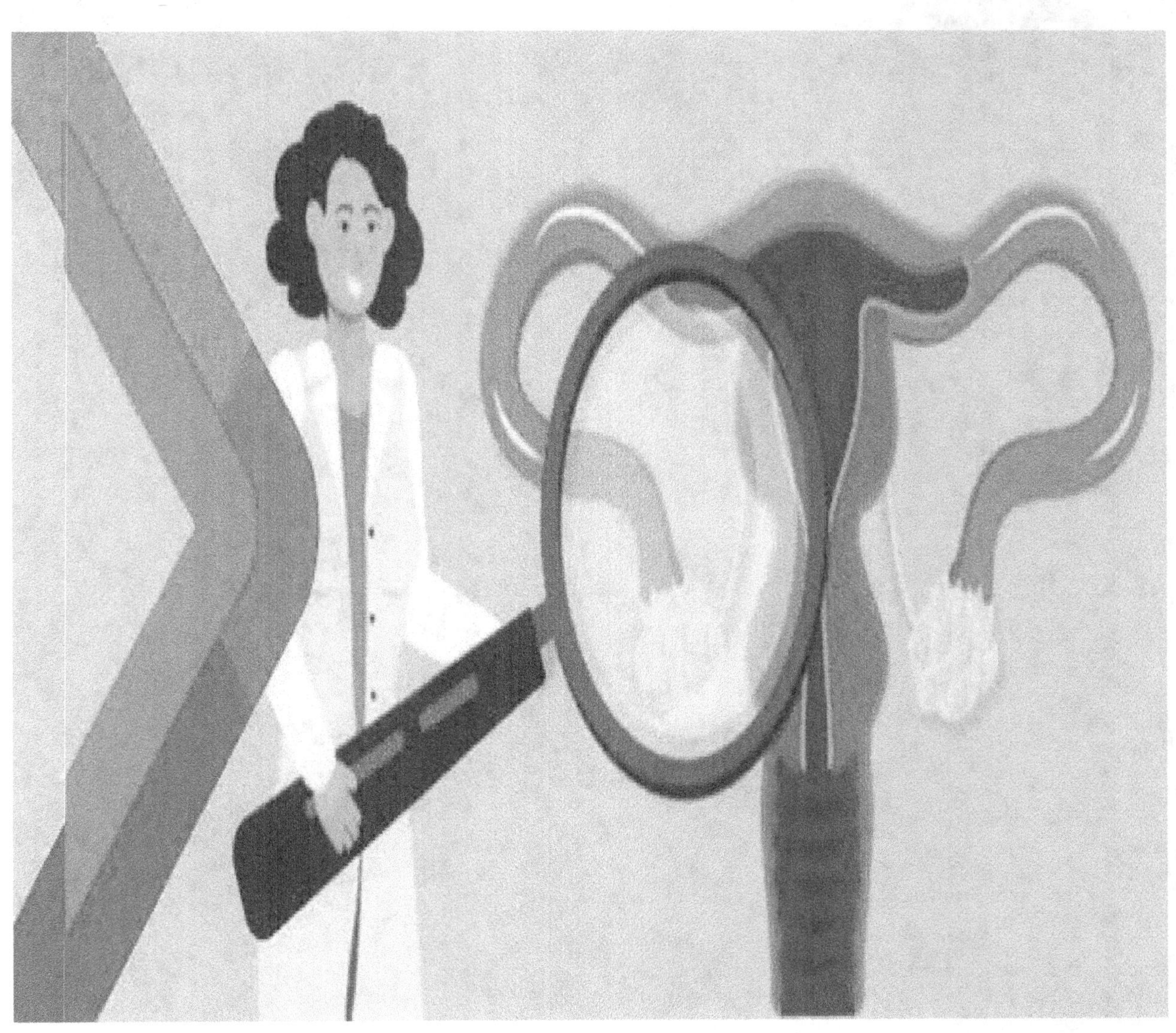

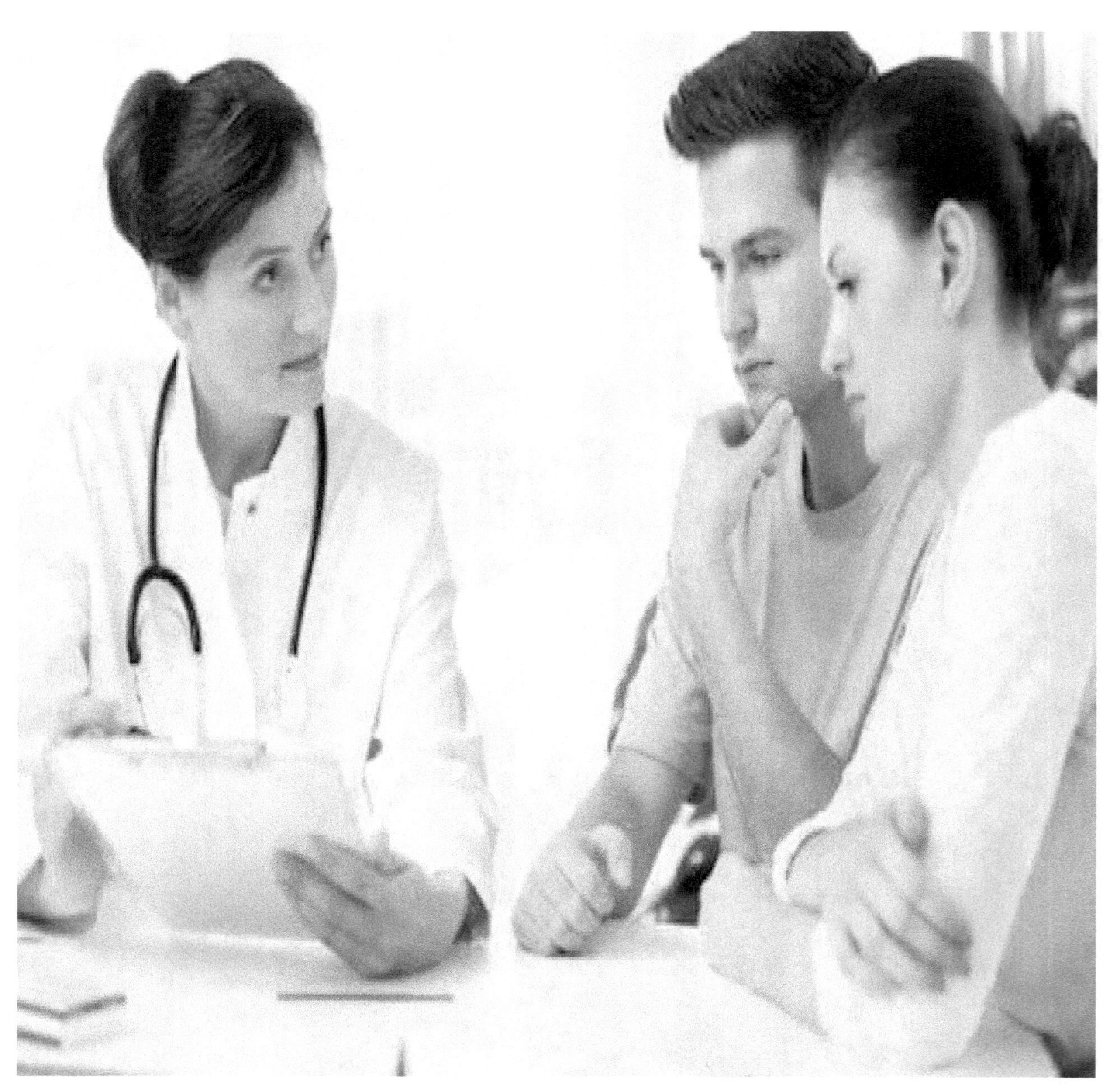

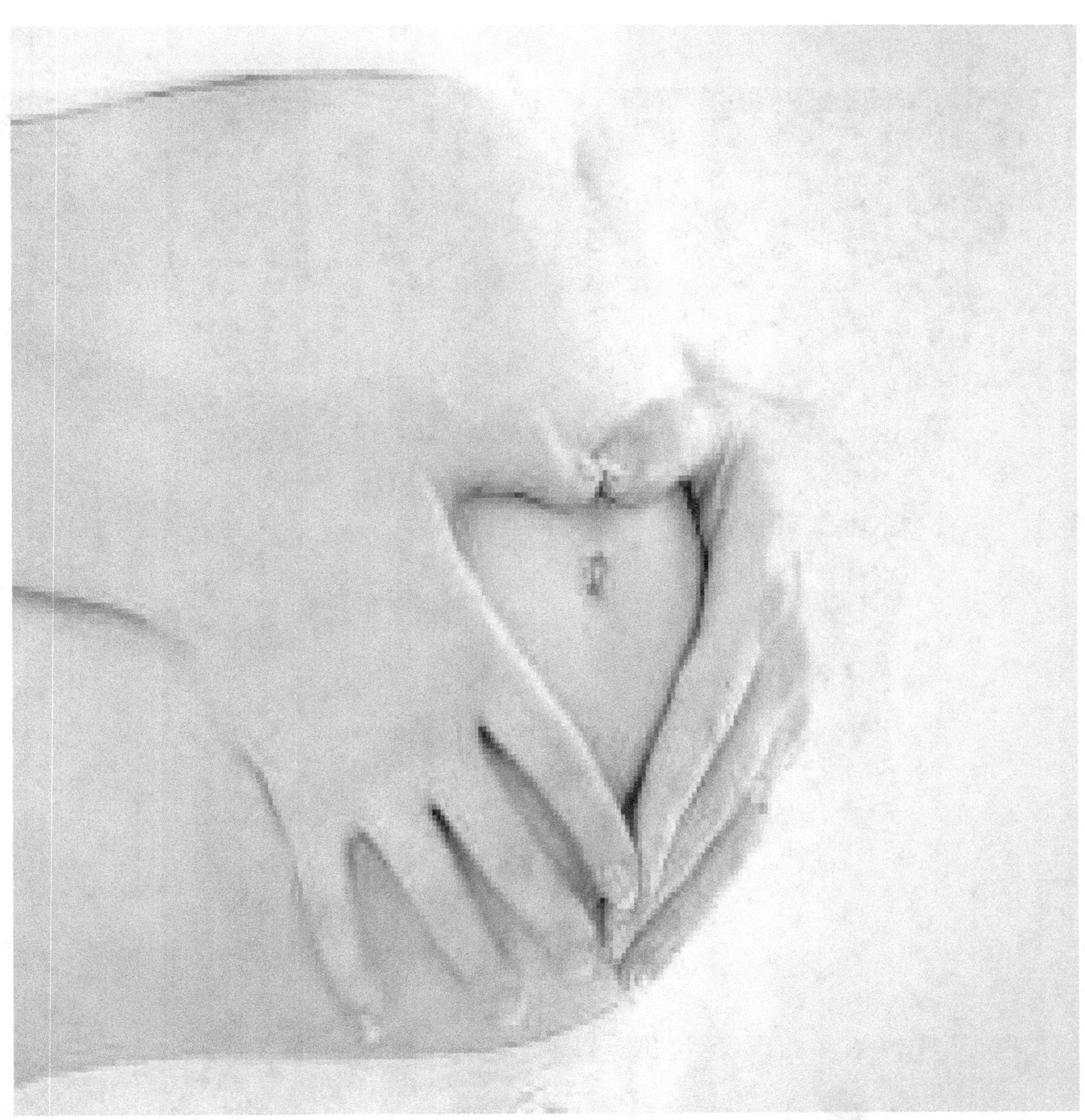

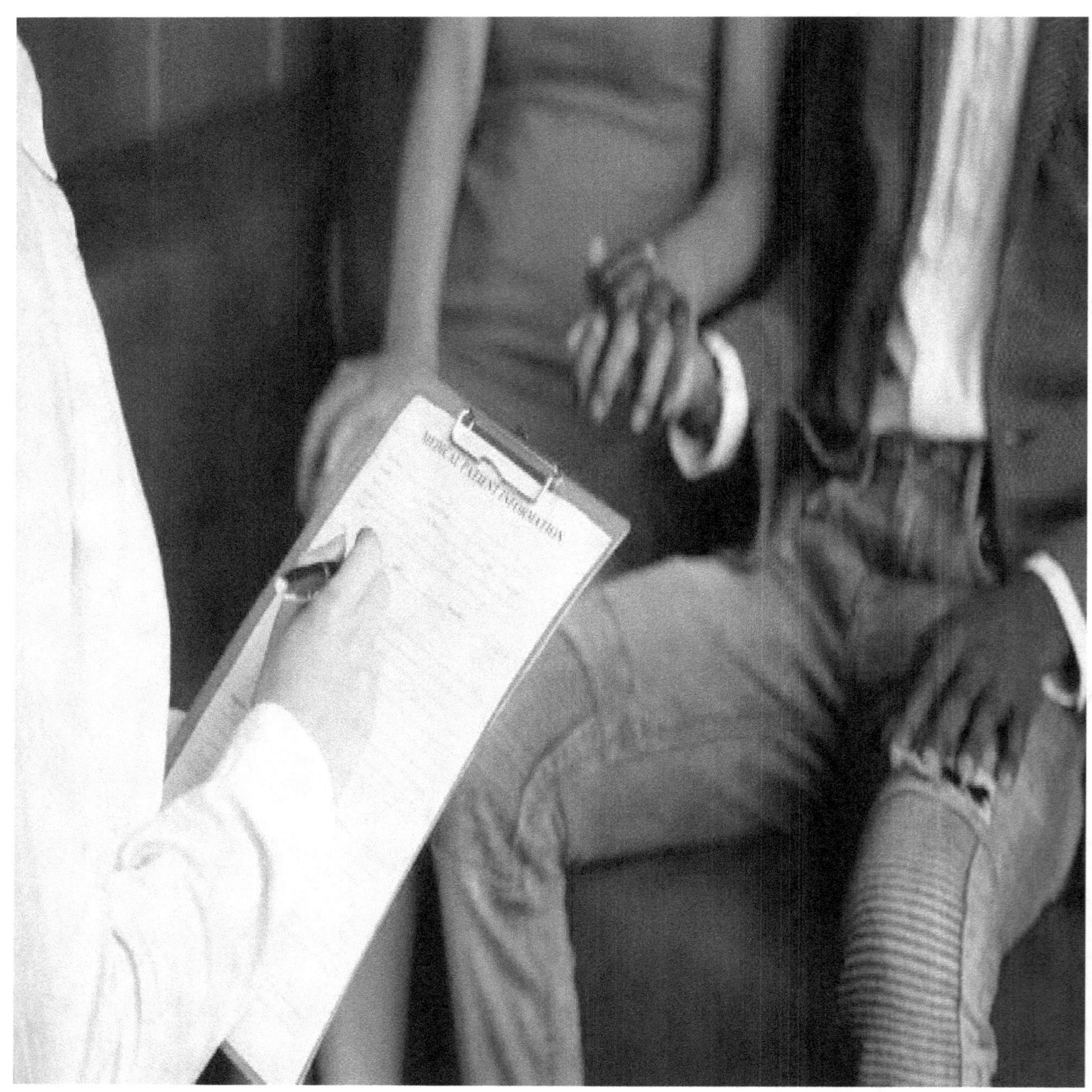

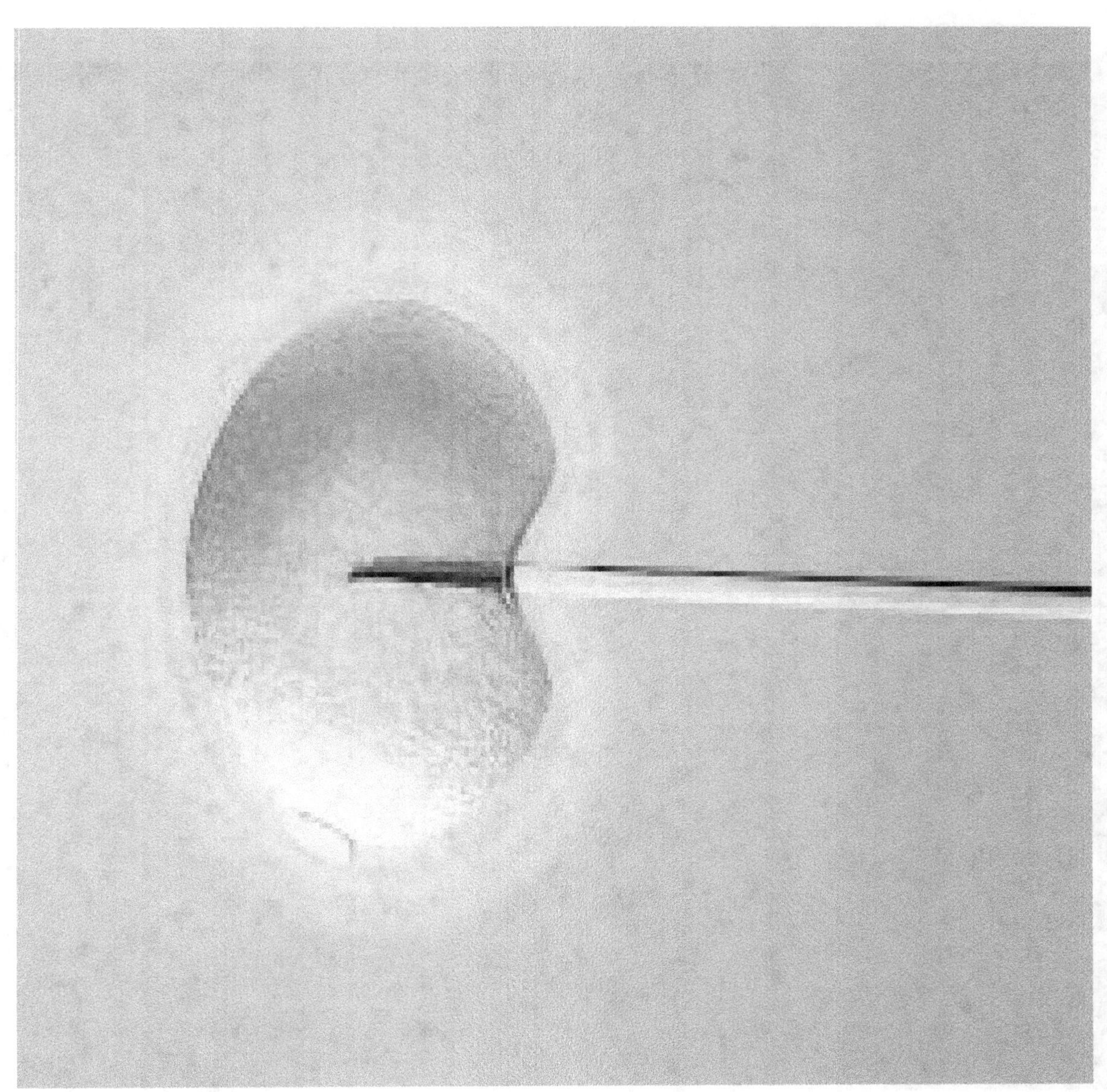

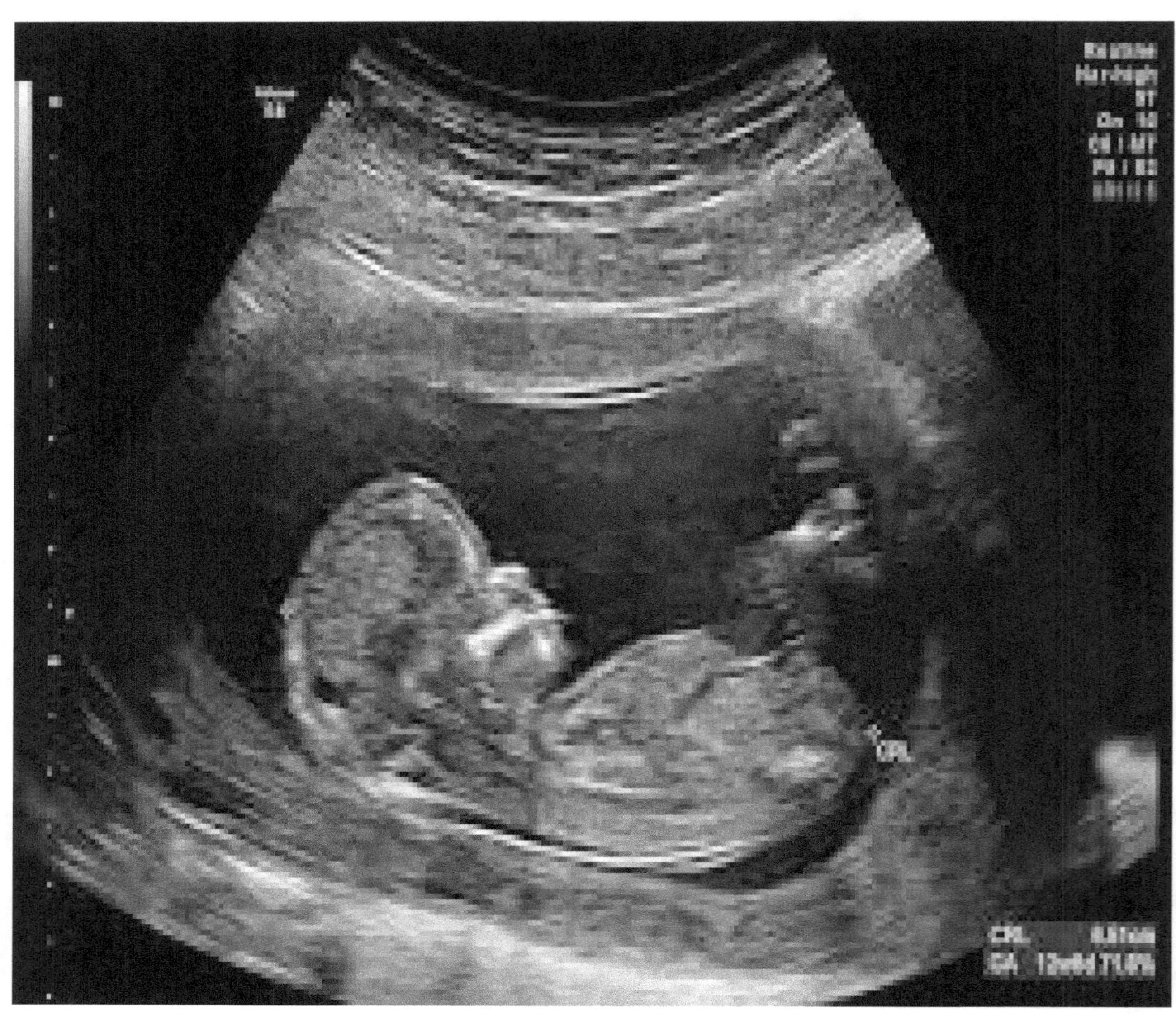